Praise and Testimonials for James and Debra Rouse and their Book

Think Eat Move Thrive

"With their latest book, the Rouses bring a refreshing and common-sense approach to making the changes necessary to living a happier, healthier, and more fulfilling life. This book is packed with common sense, wisdom, and advice and is a must read for anyone who aspires to take control of their lives in a truly life affirming way. Their holistic approach makes both intuitive and practical sense and will be truly transformational for those who follow their advice."

—**Malcolm Aylett**, financial advisor, Edward Jones

"Drs. James and Debra are the ones we often say, 'I want what they are having!' and now, they bring their wisdom, expertise, and experience to print. *Think Eat Move Thrive* is innovative, creative, and chock-full of science and inspiration. This book is written in such a way that you know the authors are right there with you, championing you onward to your most healthy self. The QR codes to the videos are fabulous. This is the companion book that supports and serves you to thrive in all areas of life."

—**Lisa Livingstone**, meeting planner, Livingstone and Associates, Denver, CO

"*Think Eat Move Thrive* is a handbook for living a healthy, happy, and fulfilled life. But more than that, it celebrates the process and possibilities around developing daily practices that allow all of us to enjoy the journey and focus less on the destination. This book will uplift and inspire you, no matter where you happen to be in life."

—**Scott Carlin**, executive/producer, SantaBu Entertainment and Soul-Centered Media

"*Think Eat Move Thrive* is inspirational and eye-opening. Drs. James and Debra have given me the confidence to care for myself and the courage to pursue my own vision of an awesome life!"

—**Brendan Harrington**, president and CEO,
Hungry Eye Media

"James Rouse is one of those very special people who can move us to rise up to our absolute best. In this powerful book, James and Debra elegantly offer us a wealth of exceptional ideas that will help anyone live the lives they've always dreamed of living."

—**Robin Sharma**, bestselling author of *The Leader Who Had No Title*
and *The Monk Who Sold His Ferrari*

"James is an amazing embodiment of body, mind, and spirit. The light and wisdom that emanate from him are extraordinary. His work is to help everyone with whom he comes into contact realize their own power and to share it with the world. I am grateful for his presence among us."

—**Reverend David Goldberg**, publisher of *Science of Mind* Magazine

"Dr. James Rouse is an amazing speaker. His ability to inspire, motivate, and be a catalyst for positive lifestyle change is unbelievable. Just being in his presence can change your life. I have worked with him since 2000 and he continues to amaze and inspire me."

—**Colleen M. Reilly**, MSM/MBA,
president of Total Well-Being, Aurora, CO

"Drs. James and Debra make optimum wellness a reality that is within every single person's reach. They are gifted at educating and truly moving people to embrace their simple yet true philosophy: we are all in charge of our thoughts and choices. Their message for all is that abundant health is our birthright and responsibility. This book offers a rousing call to action for all who desire more energy, health, and happiness."

—**Ellen Feeney**, White Wave VP Responsible Livelihood, Broomfield, CO

"There is a certain radiance that beams from Dr. James that is like the light that attracts the moth. People are drawn to him as positive energy is universally compelling or magnetic. It is the balance of relevance, humor, and depth that has a way of penetrating their psyche where they begin to ask themselves questions as they get drawn deeper into the content."

—**J. Madden**, o3consulting, owner of Pura Vida Club and Greenwood Athletic Club, Denver, CO

"After meeting Dr. James I am healthier then I have ever been, which automatically brings happiness and positive thinking. His positive energy is contagious not only for me but for everyone that has had the fortune of getting to know him. He is a real and genuine person who truly cares. I know one thing for sure, he has made me a better person not only in health but also the way I look at life in general."

—**Ken Kefalas**, CEO of Bombard Electric, Las Vegas, NV

"Dr. James has presented to my sales team twice at our National Sales Meetings. He is motivating, inspiring, educational . . . and fun! His smile, passion, and knowledge are contagious!"

—**Jane Drinkwalter**, vice president of sales,
Vitamer International, Irvine, CA

"Drs. James and Debra are lifesavers! When my doctor sounded the alarm about my high cholesterol and wanted me to begin using cholesterol-reducing drugs, I decided instead to finally and fully apply the health initiatives recommended by them. As a result, my cholesterol reverted back to excellent levels and has remained in these ranges in the years following. I have lost weight and have embraced a food and exercise regimen that has nurtured my overall health while also increasing my sense of vitality and well-being. You won't find more effective or powerful teachers in this field."

—**Dr. Roger W. Teel**, senior minister and spiritual director,
Mile Hi Church, Lakewood, CO

"Dr. James Rouse does not speak on health or wellness, he LIVES health, vitality, and wellness. He is one of the very unique people that come along and transform the lives of the audience with education and passion. James has permanently impacted my life and the lives of my employees. When he was finished speaking everyone was craving to hear more."

—**Michael Van Gilder**, CEO of Vangilder Insurance, Denver, CO

Think Eat Move Thrive

Think Eat Move Thrive

The Practice *for an* Awesome Life

Dr. James Rouse
and Dr. Debra Rouse

ATRIA BOOKS
New York London Toronto Sydney New Delhi

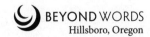
BEYOND WORDS
Hillsboro, Oregon

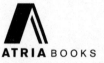

ATRIA BOOKS

A Division of Simon & Schuster, Inc.
1230 Avenue of the Americas
New York, NY 10020

BEYOND WORDS

20827 N.W. Cornell Road, Suite 500
Hillsboro, Oregon 97124-9808
503-531-8700 / 503-531-8773 fax
www.beyondword.com

The information contained in this book is intended to be educational and not for diagnosis, prescription, or treatment of any health disorder whatsoever. This information should not replace consultation with a competent healthcare professional. The content of this book is intended to be used as an adjunct to a rational and responsible healthcare program prescribed by a professional healthcare practitioner. The author and publisher are in no way liable for any misuse of the material.

Managing editor: Lindsay S. Brown
Editors: Gretchen Stelter, Emily Han
Copyeditor: Jennifer Weaver-Neist
Proofreader: Michelle Blair
Design: Devon Smith
Cover photos: Katy Moses
Composition: William H. Brunson Typography Services

First Atria Books/Beyond Words hardcover edition September 2014

ATRIA BOOKS and colophon are trademarks of Simon & Schuster, Inc. Beyond Words Publishing is an imprint of Simon & Schuster, Inc. and the Beyond Words logo is a registered trademark of Beyond Words Publishing, Inc.

For more information about special discounts for bulk purchases, please contact Simon & Schuster Special Sales at 1-866-506-1949 or business@simonandschuster.com.

The Simon & Schuster Speakers Bureau can bring authors to your live event. For more information or to book an event, contact the Simon & Schuster Speakers Bureau at 1-866-248-3049 or visit our website at www.simonspeakers.com.

Manufactured in the United States of America

10 9 8 7 6 5 4 3 2 1

Library of Congress Cataloging-in-Publication Data

Rouse, James
  Think eat move thrive : reclaim your awesome self for your best and longest life / Dr. James Rouse and Dr. Debra Rouse.
    pages   cm
Includes bibliographical references.
  1. Health—Popular works.   2. Nutrition—Popular works.   3. Physical fitness—Popular works.   4. Self-care, Health—Popular works.   I. Rouse, Debra.   II. Title.
RA776.R772   2014
613.2—dc23

                                                                        2014012566

  ISBN: 978-1-58270-492-0
  ISBN: 978-1-4767-6997-4 (ebook)

The corporate mission of Beyond Words Publishing, Inc.: *Inspire to Integrity*

For Dakota Sunshine and Elli Grace.
Our love for you fuels our pursuit of awesome living

The key to getting started down the path of being
remarkable in anything is to simply act with
the intention of being remarkable.

—**Chad Fowler**

CONTENTS

CONTENTS

CONTENTS

FOREWORD

Please know this: you are not an encapsulated bag of skin dragging around a dreary little ego; you are an evolutionary wonder—a trillion cells singing together in a vast chorale, an organism environment, a symbiosis of cell and soul. Our brains are stargates, and our bodies are celled of mysteries that invite us to enter into a Larger Body, a richer field of Mind, and a Spirit that comprehends them all. This means, however, that one agrees to relinquish those limited and limiting patterns of body (sensory and motor); of emotion; of volition; of intelligence and understanding; of spirit; and of the lazy daily practice of thinking, eating, and moving that have been keeping you from becoming all that you can be. Allow yourself to instead become available to the extraordinary dimensions that each of us contain for much larger life in body, mind, and spirit.

Once in a long while, a book and teaching comes along that addresses this challenge while providing state-of-the-art knowledge for achieving a life of excellence. The authors, Drs. James and Debra Rouse, know the powers of which they teach. Indeed, they give full warning of what can be expected:

FOREWORD

This book is designed to make you uncomfortable, push many of your buttons, and get you to leave most, if not all, of your old self behind. . . . From this moment forward, commit to being a student of creating the very best life. Open your mind to new thoughts and visions for living, giving, and feeling. Open your body to being a force of strength, beauty, grace, and limitless energy. Open your spirit to being peaceful, grateful, courageous, and loving. Your life purpose is to realize your highest expression; this is your time.

Brave words, but an outcome that is entirely possible, as shown in the precise but potent training given in these pages. You, the committed reader, will truly emerge from the cocoon of old ways of being in following the plan for complete life change. You will eat differently, move beautifully, think on many planes, and above all, *Thrive!*

—Jean Houston, author of *The Wizard of Us*

PREFACE

This book contains "the practice" for daily living that is as simple as it is powerful. The daily practice of Think, Eat, Move, when mindfully and proactively integrated and embraced into your life, will support you in creating and experiencing your "greatest day" everyday.

Dr. James's Story

As a wellness and lifestyle expert and a baby boomer at midlife, I have made it my professional and personal mission to take a stand and not fall prey to what many see as the inevitable decline and demise of our collective health, vitality, and outlook as a nation. This in spite of the challenging facts, daunting statistics, and what appears to be a direct and downward trend toward greater doom and gloom in regard to the health and well-being of Americans. I know that we are better than these facts and figures, and that we, as a collective whole, are ready to reverse the trends in obesity, diabetes, cancer, depression, and self-imposed malaise.

My optimism is growing; I see powerful reasons for hope. I hear it from friends and strangers, from schools and communities, from neighbors, and from professional colleagues. I see it in the way people desire to be more, to be better—to catch fire again and reclaim the life and livelihood they came here to express. By taking responsibility and applying the simple, empowering, and revolutionary principles found in this book, you will not only transform your health and well-being but also your overall happiness and life fulfillment. As a result, you will act as a catalyst to shift the tides, the momentum, and the grim outlook of those around you. Indeed, these interesting times will require transformation of our self-imposed mediocrity in order to build a movement toward outstanding, awesome, and epic world-class living.

I know personally how it feels to transform a life from average to amazing. I did not grow up in a highly functional, optimistic, exercise-focused, and veggie-and-granola-eating family; and I know what it is like to face one's mortality. I have loved and lost parents, friends, and patients to preventable diseases. I have sat with Buddhist monks at 20,000 feet in the Himalayas and worked the graveyard shift at truck stops. I have experienced generations of alcoholism and thrived living in a spiritual community. I have built and lost multimillion-dollar businesses; and I have been brought to my knees with a learning disability and a love for the human spirit and God.

•   •   •   •

My life today is a very different experience than the beginning of my life. My genetic heritage is scarred by cancer, diabetes, heart disease, alcoholism, and depression; and my early years were marked by fear and stress. But my parents had tenacity and grit, which has been a blessing to me along my journey; they loved me but struggled together. My self-esteem and confidence suffered, and I struggled in school with dyslexia and barely graduated high school. I was constantly beating myself up, finding fault, and replacing what I perceived as criticism and disappointment with my own version of self-loathing.

My early teen years were a time of great struggle. One morning, I stayed home from school, faking being sick because I was too scared to take a math test. The combination of being challenged with undiagnosed dyslexia and suffering from low confidence made for severe test anxiety. This particular morning, Jack LaLanne entered our living room via his television show. Decked out in his signature blue jumpsuit, I was mesmerized by his energy and his desire to serve and inspire. I could not take my eyes off him! Jack said that daily exercise was the penance that he paid for being able to feel good all day long. Boy, was I ready to feel good! I bought into every single word he said, and in that moment, Jack became my teacher and my mentor. He was exactly what I wanted and needed in my life; he tapped something deep inside me, and I was forever changed.

"All motion creates positive emotion," said Jack. At that time, I did not fully understand the power of movement—how it positively affects psychology, giving one the ability to navigate stress in a healthier way; its power to raise self-esteem, confidence, brilliance, and presence. Today, I absolutely live by this motto. I strive to be a testament to it daily, and there is no doubt that it saved my life—and it will do the same for you.

My love of movement and mindfulness led me to study many other great teachers of self-development. From meditation to yoga to mysticism, I began to devour it all. I coupled my physical development and growth with the study of holistic health and well-being by integrating Eastern and Western ideas and practices on how to achieve peak living and thriving. My deep, burning desire was to heal my wounded and defeated self, shift my paradigm from surviving to thriving, and take what I was learning and share it with the world around me.

The love of living well gave me the vision to become a physician, despite being told by my high school guidance counselor that I'd be better served at a technical school, if anywhere. College was no easy task, but I was bound and determined to succeed. It was a rough road before I finally landed at Marlboro College, a small liberal arts college in Vermont where I received my undergraduate degree. From there, I chose the holistic path of naturopathic medicine, which combines Western (conventional) medicine and science with nutrition, exercise, herbal medicine, homeopathy, acupuncture, and lifestyle medicine. Naturopathic medical school gave me a greater appreciation for science and an understanding of how the body works. The integrative, holistic philosophy opened my eyes to the idea of body and mind working together to create a life of limitless happiness, vitality, and empowerment.

Over the past twenty-plus years, I have witnessed the positive transformation of others, both professionally and personally, when they decide to become fully alive. From my experiences, this is what I know: we all have a story, and we can choose to allow this story to dictate our life's experiences—or not. We can use it as an excuse to hold us back and keep us living small, or we can use it to serve us in making our life an epic expression of *awesome*.

Dr. Debra's Story

A few years ago, I had the privilege of traveling to India with Made by Survivors, an international nonprofit organization that employs and educates survivors of slavery and other human rights abuses, including women and children living in red-light areas and border towns in extreme poverty. I had the honor of working with young women who had been victims of trafficking and sex slavery, and it was a life-changing, transformational experience for me on so many levels. These young women had lived through hell but were now living in shelter homes of safety, restoration, and rehabilitation, receiving the necessary support, education, nutrition, and love that had been taken from them at an early age—some as young as nine and ten years old. They were learning many life skills for the first time, including self-empowerment and self-love.

These girls had so much hope and love and joy in their hearts, in spite of the unspeakable horrors they experienced in their young lives. I witnessed this firsthand when I had the chance to talk to a group of survivors about self-care, nutrition, their bodies, and what it means to have a positive body image. I'm not sure why I was expecting something different, but I was surprised that they wanted the same things most of us want—to feel beautiful, loved, strong, and safe. They didn't feel sorry for themselves, blame their circumstances, or dwell on their past experiences. Instead, they looked boldly ahead at what they were becoming, and were grateful every day for the opportunity to learn and grow.

What if we all approached life and our self-care with such appreciation, enthusiasm, and intention? I truly believe that self-care is a form of social activism; it is not selfish. It is the means through which we can transform ourselves and those around us.

It is my deepest desire to effect change in the mental, emotional, physical, and spiritual health of individuals and communities across our country and globally. As a natural optimist, I can admit that it sometimes makes me sad when I experience beautiful, talented, and gifted beings self-sabotaging by buying into the idea that they'll never be happy, fit, loved, successful, or healthy because it's just not in the cards for them this lifetime. I don't buy it. We're all here to make a difference; and we're all deserving and capable of loving relationships, radiant health, and happiness.

Since my experience in India, I believe I won the life lottery by being born in North America during a time when, for the most part, I am free to do, create, and be anything that I desire. I haven't always made the best choices, but every moment of every day I can choose to do something differently. I am free. I am worthy and so are you—I want you to know that deep within your soul. I want you to know that you are loved.

More important than anything else is the idea that despite your history or my history, past or present, we are here to do something great—to thrive. It is my mission to share what I know with you and others so that you can experience more happiness, peace, and love in your life and then spread it across the nation and the world. I believe in you—that your own personal mission and vision are necessary on this planet, which is why your self-care is so important.

• • • •

Both James and I are excited to share our experience and our expertise with you. We hope you will use some of our practices of positive and proactive thinking; mindful, healthy, and plant-based eating; and moving daily to claim or reclaim your awesome self in order to thrive.

Do it for yourself, those you love, and those you've never even met. The world will be better and brighter, and so will you.

Namaste.

INTRODUCTION

My life is my message.
—**His Holiness the Dalai Lama**

Take a look around you and notice what level of health, happiness, vitality, and fulfillment you see. World Health Organization (WHO) research states that one out of every three Americans is depressed, and the United States is ranked second in the world for the highest rates of depression (France is ranked number one). The WHO estimates 350 million people worldwide are affected by depression.[1] Type 2 diabetes, heart disease, obesity, and other diseases of choice in lifestyle are all on the rise as well. At this time in the United States, nearly 70 percent of adults (69.2 percent, according to the Centers for Disease Control) are overweight or obese.[2] We, as a country, are not sleeping well, and less than 20 percent of us report that we are satisfied with our jobs.[3]

The healthcare system really isn't a "health"-care system at all. Rather, it is a disease-care system that is not built to support, educate, or inspire well-being. In the year 2011, global spending for pharmaceutical drugs topped $950 billion, and the United States accounts for over half of that spending.[4] We can't help but fantasize about how things could be different if that money went toward education, prevention, and inspiring people to take charge of their health. The more we become tethered to pharmaceutical companies and managed care, the more disempowered and disconnected we are from our true source of vitality, peace, and joy. Our collective confidence is waning; and we appear to be more vulnerable than ever to losing our battle with complacency, mediocrity, and inflammation.

We're living at a time when inflammation, in our bodies and brains, is leading to a host of chronic diseases from which we are dying: diabetes, cancer, Alzheimer's, depression, and obesity. Our attitude and our outlook on life is a main driver for whether or not inflammation becomes an issue for us (along with healthy exercise and diet).

The vast majority of our nation is overweight, sad, tired, stressed out, and underliving. People have forgotten how good they are and have bought into the myth that there is some sort of physiological conspiracy keeping them from living the life of their dreams. The planet is in need of an all-out self-care revolution, and it begins with three essential and basic ingredients: THINK, EAT, and MOVE.

When the body is not performing or looking the way we desire it to, we tend to focus on diet or both diet and exercise. Or we may choose the route of therapy and work on our mental and emotional issues. Each of these individual actions can be empowering and support growth and healing. However, when you marry and optimize the practices of mindfulness, eating with intention, and interval-based movement, you will witness a complete transformation—you will Thrive.

Your Complete Life Wellness

Think Eat Move Thrive (TEMT) builds a foundation for complete life wellness: it's all about creating a revolution from within. The revolution is an evolution from drug and reactive care to loving, empowered, and proactive self-care. To date, most diets and self-improvement programs focus on losing weight, getting ripped, or other goals that only lead to short-term happiness. If we want long-lasting, inspired change, the driving motivator needs to be intrinsic in nature—as easy and natural as breathing. If we can identify the source of our inspiration and set new, deep-seated intentions for health, wellness, and happiness, we can actively move forward and integrate our goals into our daily lives. The wonderful side effects are feeling greater vitality, joy, confidence, and longevity. Again, the simple recipe is integrating three basic fundamentals: Think, Eat, and Move.

- Think: cultivating mindfulness and empowering attitudes shifts our limiting beliefs and habits;
- Eat: eating with intention fuels our minds for greater clarity and our bodies for greater performance;
- Move: participating in interval-based movement, resistance training—any fitness-inspired activity—and natural incidental movement strengthens our bodies inside and out for complete fitness, lasting results, and greater longevity.

The integration of these core ingredients helps us Thrive. What we've seen over and over again is that when we thrive and care for ourselves with love, we become a powerful source for social activism. When we perform at our best, we also best serve our families, friends, coworkers, communities, and the world. It's beautiful to see what this kind of personal intention can manifest.

The world needs our examples of inspired living. Realizing your best life is not only about looking good, it's also about inspiring others around you to realize their best lives. When one of us decides to truly step up and own our life from the inside out, everyone around us is elevated. When you dedicate yourself to becoming your best, others are inspired to do the same. When you choose to show up and take a stand for love, to be courageous, and to live your life with purpose and passion, you cannot help but lift the world around you. When you do this, you become an agent of change.

The Book

The book is divided into three parts: THINK, EAT, MOVE. Within each of these first three parts, there are chapters that go deeper into different aspects of each practice, providing scientific facts and personal stories that explain their individual importance and impact. At the end of each chapter, there is an exercise to help you put that idea into action and confidently develop rituals of awareness and thriving for years to come. As you move through each section and rebuild the fundamentals of thinking, eating, and moving, you will notice how each part leads into and expands upon the others. We recommend that you take the time to read through each part in order, and then feel free to go back to specific areas, jumping around as needed to those areas that you want to focus on.

Since this is a book by two people—with two sets of expertise, experiences, and ideas—you'll see check-ins from each of us where we think our unique perspective could add something to your understanding. You'll also see short action steps throughout the chapters, to provide you with quick, easy, immediate practices.

There are also QR tags—snappy online links—that provide bonus content for a multimedia experience. You can watch us do exercises and check out how to whip up James's favorite pancakes. The idea is to give you the most rewarding and personal experience possible as you use this book as your personal guide. We highly recommend that you have a journal in which you can take notes along the way. You may want to jot down ideas or thoughts that come up for you (and some action steps call for this), or you may want to use it as a place to write down answers to some of the questions we pose.

Our appendices are intended to give you the tools needed to implement this life of thriving. We want you to be psyched for this journey and excited to continue the journey as a life-long learner. We've tried to anticipate questions that may come up along the way and trust you will find the answers you are looking for within these pages.

The TEMT Program

At the end of the book is our 30-day program to put TEMT into action. The TEMT meal plan challenges the status quo and our Standard American Diet (SAD). The fundamental difference is that SAD is predominately comprised of convenience foods, processed and packaged foods, an overload of sugar and salt, unhealthy fats, and too many calories; whereas the TEMT plan focuses on anti-inflammatory foods, lifestyle, and longevity. This program offers simple, science-based solutions that address not just the causes but the beliefs and mindsets that have created this epidemic of unhappiness, unhealthiness, and underliving. TEMT will help prevent many of the diseases associated with inflammation through the practices of optimizing our thinking, eating, and moving.

Our wellness is about more than what our bodies look like (especially in comparison to the cultural and social ideals of the media). True wellness is about fueling our bodies with the right foods while also nurturing our minds and keeping them active. It is about moving daily so we maintain a healthy mind and body as much as it's about staying limber, fit, and strong. Our wellness is about thriving from the inside out.

The 30-day TEMT Program speaks to the idea that happiness and a thriving life isn't a destination, it's a daily practice. The daily practice comes through right thinking, mindful eating, and consistently moving, which translates to thriving every single day. This is the essence of our book; and with our TEMT Program, we are going to help you create the discipline and the proper chemistry to work these three principles into a daily practice.

Our Promise

Why do most diets fail, and why do many self-help programs fail to deliver? Because they don't get into real-life, practical details—the heart of what we do all day long, every day. Nor do they take into consideration our whole beings—bodies, minds, and spirits—instead focusing on fragmented parts that need to be "fixed." In contrast, TEMT offers you an inspiring, science-based map for how to live your best and fullest life day by day.

This book is designed to make you uncomfortable, push many of your buttons, and get you to leave most, if not all, of your old self behind. From this point forward, commit to letting go of anything that is not presently serving you—guilt, jealousy, perfectionism, regret, fear of failure or success. From this moment forward, commit to being a student of creating the very best life. Open your mind to new thoughts and visions for living, giving, and feeling. Open your body to being a force of strength, beauty, grace, and limitless energy. Open your spirit to being peaceful, grateful, courageous, and loving. Your life purpose is to realize your highest expression; this is your time.

This is a book and program about self-mastery and self-love. TEMT is not just a lifestyle, it is a life study. Do the work, commit to your self-care and self-love, and you will hold the keys to reinventing, reclaiming, and reframing not only your life but also the lives of everyone around you.

Age, religion, socioeconomic status, politics, race, and gender are irrelevant here. No matter where or who you are in life, you will benefit from these practices and principles.

We're honored you've decided to make time for yourself and include us in your journey. Let's create a wellness revolution through empowered thinking, clean eating, and daily movement. Together, let's THRIVE.

 Welcome from Dr. James and Dr. Debra:
http://www.youtube.com/watch?v=8GrHjKj80_Y&feature=youtu. be

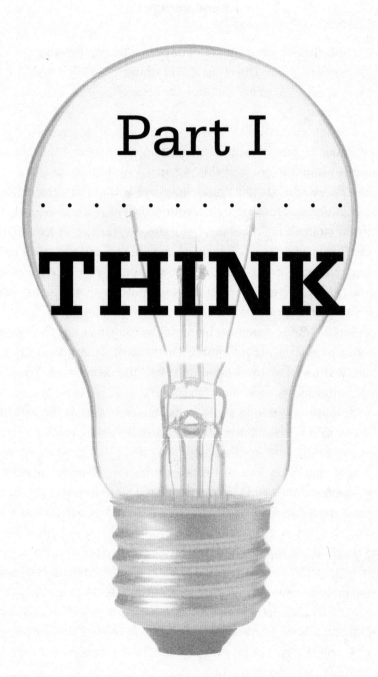

Part I

THINK

Part I: THINK

All that we are is the result of what we have thought.
The mind is everything.
What we think we become.

—Buddha

In general, as human beings, we settle for the status quo that surrounds us, and because of this, we may not be fully satisfied with the way things are, whether these things are within our personal lives (jobs, relationships, income level, health, looks) or in the larger scope of our world (state of the economy, homelessness, hunger, environment). We can accept that "this is how it is" and think we're powerless to do anything about it. If our thinking is the impetus of what creates our experience, what happens when our thoughts are that of being powerless and even hopeless? Would this mean we are content to live a life of mediocrity? If the power of thought is transformational then we are proposing to you the idea of joining a movement against mediocrity by looking at the way we think about our lives and our actions. When we change our thinking, we change our lives.

Assuming every action and every outcome begins as thought, this section—THINK—is about cultivating mindfulness and empowering attitudes that will shift limiting thoughts, beliefs, and habits from average to amazing. What does that mean specifically? It means we need to know how our brains and thinking works, so we can effectively change our patterns and be intrinsically motivated to change our current state.

The chapters in this section are all about helping to build a better brain chemistry to support high-level wellness, peak performance, optimism, happiness, and motivation. We build great thinking and decision making through awareness and intention—two essential ingredients that are integral to thriving. Thoughts can manifest into action, and doing mindfulness practices throughout the day to keep our thinking positive and clear will optimize all areas of your life. To effect positive change, the first step is Think, so let's dive in!

THINK

 Consider the Power of Thought:
http://youtu.be/SLShW6gAeY0

1

THINK Change

A book like this is read for one main reason: the desire to change and to grow—to create a life of greater meaning, success, and happiness. But it's not always easy. In fact, it's almost never easy. If it were, we'd be able to do it with minimal help and at the drop of a hat. In reality, even small changes can take a long time and diligent, dedicated work. You've taken the first step; you picked up this book and decided you want to change. Now it's time to look at the mental blocks that come with change.

Become a Change Agent

Why is it so many of us do the same thing over and over again and expect different results? Many have simply called this insanity. Most of us have been stuck at some point in our lives. We want to feel better, look better, experience more love and connection in relationships, but we don't change any of our behaviors and end up spinning our wheels. Forget changing others. Nothing changes if we don't do the work to change ourselves. Sometimes things may get so bad that we feel as if we'll never emerge from the darkness we've created for ourselves; it can be overwhelming. And as painful as our current comfort zone may feel, getting outside of it—taking a leap of faith—can seem excruciating.

So, how do we change? How do we train our brains to build a new groove and pave our life paths with passion and purpose?

You can start by taking a thoughtful look at your life. Study your daily paradigm and compassionately examine the patterns that you have adopted or cemented into habits. Ask yourself:

- Are these habits taking you to the level of livingness that you desire?
- Will you experience the life that you dream of if you stay the present course?
- If you choose to follow your current train of thought and actions, will you fulfill your life purpose and fully realize the gifts that you have been given?
- How do you stop doing the same thing over and over again and start enacting real change?

We love comfort; our brains are literally wired for it. We are wired to stay where we are and seek out what is convenient. We may call this living in the "comfort zone" or "being in a rut," or even "insanity." Whatever we label it, it will get us nowhere in life. It takes a big vision, a compelling *why* to get us to move out of our own way and begin moving toward our highest expression—in spite of feeling uncomfortable!

Author Check-In

James's *why*: I have found my *why* to be a combination of things. Spiritually, I am wired to serve—sharing my passion for personal discovery and development, for body and mind performance, and for life transformation. This drives me to set "stretch goals" every day—to learn and be more than the day before and to show up and grow for the people I love the most, my family.

Debra's *why*: Similar to James, my *why* is driven by my desire to serve and show up in life fully alive, energized, optimistic, healthy, and engaged (for myself, my family, and my friends). I am motivated by life itself and by my wish to see, touch, and experience new adventures—to challenge myself mentally and physically and never take for granted my God-given gifts. My two daughters are my most powerful *whys*. Not because my life is solely focused on them, but because I want to lead by examples so that they witness a life of full engagement, and what they take away from my examples is that they are infinitely capable of creating the life of their dreams.

Many of us want to believe that success can happen overnight, whether that comes through a pill, a lover, or a new pair of shoes. The media and advertising companies take full advantage of this desire. We need to stop the cycle of buying quick-fix products and hoping for a magical cure. As much as we might hate to admit it, we like conformity; most of us are content doing the things that are expected of us, not much more or less. We set our expectations at a certain level and that becomes our acceptable standard.

Powerful and sustainable change—the real, lasting kind—only happens with consistent work on the fundamentals. Doing things well day in and day out creates the new paradigm, laying the foundation for a thriving life. Highly successful and fulfilled people consistently show up for life; they make commitments and they keep them. They manage their time and practice the habits they want to make their own. These are things that usually happen behind the glossy scenes of success. They are not necessarily sexy or glamorous, yet these are the things that are done again and again, creating a life of success, effectiveness, freedom, creativity, and integrity over time. Daily habits become rituals, which are the tenets of success and the basis for peace, power, and purpose. We like to use the idea of "bookending" our days to help set us up for success.

Bookending

Bookends are a simple way of structuring your day to allow for growth and recovery. The morning bookend is the Hour of Power. This one habit will rock everything around you—increase your energy, optimism, metabolism, brilliance, creativity, production, drive, success, overall life fulfillment, and a whole lot more.

Here is what it looks like:

1. Set the intention and the alarm clock to get up and out of bed before sunrise (or at least by 5:00 AM).
2. Take care of your personal hygiene and private business before meditating for ten to twenty minutes.
3. Visualize and affirm your goals and intentions; see them as done and be grateful ahead of time. This should take about ten minutes.
4. Now it's time for exercise and movement: a combination of interval-based cardio, strength and resistance training, yoga, stretching—anything that engages your energy and your heart. Note: this can be done in thirty minutes or less. (There's more in the MOVE section on this.)
5. Breakfast—do not skip this step. Include a balance of protein, healthy fats, and fiber from fruits, veggies, and/or whole grains. (See the EAT section for more on this.)

At the end of the day, another bookend, Relaxation Rituals, is placed to signal a time-out and an official conclusion to your day. This may look like sipping a calming cup of chamomile tea, reading, stretching, or journaling.

We do not do our best work at night, especially when we have been at it all day. We do our best work when we are fresh in mind and body. For us, bookending our day means being with family and loved ones, being quiet, being still—immersing ourselves in uplifting reading and being in gratitude for the day we have just lived.

Your bookends will allow you to cultivate wisdom along with healthy sleep chemistry. They will become a ritual and a live demonstration of the love and faith you have in yourself, and everything and everyone around you.

We are surrounded by what appears to be instant gratification, but in truth, anything that is truly magnificent is created by the daily discipline of doing what needs to be done. We have to be willing to move beyond complacency and mediocrity.

This work will ask everything of you. It will ask you to step outside your comfort zone. It will ask you to show up and be present for the life that you are building one choice, one thought, and one action at a time. When you string together a series of good actions and decisions, you will see your life transform and your confidence rise, and you will be on fire with purpose and passion.

• • • • • • • • • • • •

ACTION STEP

Our dear friend, inspirational speaker, hypnotherapist, and officiant at our wedding, Jody Stevenson, recently shared this powerful affirmation at a talk she gave at Mile Hi Church in Denver, Colorado.[1] It comes from Tao wisdom. If you like it and it works for you, we suggest you repeat it aloud, in the mirror, every morning and every evening. Otherwise, feel free to come up with your own words of inspiration, or read a quote that brings inspiration to your heart:

I come from greatness.
I allow greatness.
I am greatness.

•   •   •   •   •   •   •   •   •   •   •   •

Are You Coming from Love?

Sometimes life will encourage and at other times it will force you to do this tough work—this work that is deep and at times challenging but is always done in the name of love. Each change you try to make can be made more effective when you ask, "Am I coming from love?" or "What would love do now?"

The Power of Words

As you navigate your day, practice paying attention to your words when you speak to others. Words are powerful. Are you using uplifting and empowering words toward yourself and life in general? What are the first words that you use upon waking in the morning? The words that you use will create the way you feel and set the tone for the minutes, hours, and days that follow. This is a powerful, proactive contemplation that will enable you to witness how your words can quite literally cast a spell on yourself, your actions, and maybe even on the actions of the people around you.

These questions asked silently throughout your daily living will bring clarity, power, and purpose to every action and decision, and bring greater peace to your life. When you come from love, you come from a place of wholeness—a place of service. Here are a few examples: Are you coming from love when you make a comment on someone's Facebook post? Are you asking yourself *What would love do?* when your spouse forgets an important item on the grocery list? When we stop and reflect on these questions before we react, everyone benefits.

Ask yourself this question before you choose what you will be eating, for example. When you choose a bag of chips or some other refined food that isn't good for you, you will know if it is about feeding an emotion; feeding stress; feeding an old, worn-out belief or wound. Ask yourself, *Would I eat this if I were coming from love?* When we come from love, it slows down the pace of our mind and life to be present; it calls us to stand in integrity!

Similarly, we can ask this question when we are interacting with our friends, spouse, children, and coworkers. Coming from a place of love prior to confronting a potentially uncomfortable situation helps balance the emotions that often go on overdrive and become reactionary during such confrontations.

· · · · · · · · · · · ·

ACTION STEP

A powerful way to keep this practice moving in your life is to use every doorway and threshold to remind you to show up heart first, coming from love. Each and every day, you will literally pass through many doorways. For example, the first thing in the morning, you likely pass from your bedroom to the bathroom, then another doorway into your kitchen, and more throughout the day—many times. Use these doorways as reminders to come into each new space from a mindset of love.

The practice of coming from love gives you presence of mind, presence of body, and presence of Spirit. Affirm dozens of times daily: "Come from love." And experience your happiness growing. Notice how your personal practice will inspire and uplift others.

· · · · · · · · · · · ·

Change Becomes You

We are happiest when we are working toward a goal that comes from love—one we deem worthwhile, one that we feel is important enough to dedicate daily discipline to, and one that makes us slightly uncomfortable. We are happier when we stretch ourselves to do things that take us just beyond our comfort zone; comfort just makes us lazy. When we regularly stretch our minds, bodies, and spirits, we invite possibility and inspiration. This represents a great and empowering challenge, as we will need to shift our paradigm in order to become our highest selves. In this daily work lies true and irrevocable happiness.

We are big fans of using the power of beliefs to help support any and all growth initiatives, including making changes. Beliefs can be seen as the windows you look through to see the world. You must believe that making a change is something that will help you; you must believe you will be successful. You must believe that change—no matter how uncomfortable or painful it feels at first—is in your highest interest.

Look at your present existence. Understand that most of the everyday excuses we give for not wanting or fearing change come from old habits, not fear of actual dangers. Once you tame and reprogram these false beliefs that you have about change, and see that change is all about being and having *more*—more growth, more power, more living—you will know that you are ready to truly begin. Change will become something that you look forward to and embrace.

• • • • • • • • • • • •

ACTION STEP

What changes do you need to make in order to grow? Where could you make an upgrade in your environment to support yourself? What questions can you ask yourself right now to wake up from your self-imposed slumber of mediocrity? Courageously answer these questions in a way that lights a fire in your heart and moves you to do all that is necessary to change, grow, and become all that you came here to be.

Now, look within yourself and discover your *why*.

1. What makes you excited?
2. Who inspires you?
3. What are three specific areas of your life that you are committed to changing?
4. What are your three most powerful *whys* related to these areas?

Write your responses to these questions in your notebook or journal so you can reference them later. They will not only deliver awesome and life-changing results, they will also help you align with your *why*, delivering on the promises that you came here to fulfill: to serve, inspire, create, and leave a legacy of meaning and full-on love and livingness.

• • • • • • • • • • • •

 Close the Gap to Transform Your Life:
http://www.youtube.com/watch?v=vZRIjbZOIJU&list=PLDF2
6DC5254801299

Intrinsic Versus Extrinsic Motivation

Genuine motivation is intrinsic in nature. Intrinsic motivation is driven by love (of self and others), self-improvement, self-mastery, purpose, and service; it comes from within and is impelled by a genuine interest in the goal or mission itself. You may find it helpful to think of intrinsic motivation as coming from your heart rather than coming from your ego. The TEMT plan keeps us intrinsically motivated because it is a comprehensive plan that helps balance every aspect of our lives, thus creating lasting change. We created it from a place of intrinsic motivation.

When you are motivated from your own sense of purpose and passion, you will have more energy and be more committed to staying inspired daily. In the business world, it has been shown that employees perform better and sustain long-term motivation when the work has deeper meaning. Most people are more motivated to work harder and reach goals more often for intrinsic safisfaction and meaning than they are for money. The same can be said of any goals that you may have around weight loss, exercise, or eating well. All of these goals are more likely to be actualized when they are connected to something deeply felt and more significant than a new dress size, a number on the scale, or how many *oohs* and *ahhs* you get at your high school reunion.

These extrinsic goals, as good as they feel to your ego, tend to be short-lived. That is one of the many reasons that we typically do not stay on our diets and give up our exercise programs. SAD (Standard American Diet) is easy to slide back into because it gives us a false sense of comfort; it's what we're used to. After our desire to look good or complete that 5K is fulfilled, our courage to step out of the comfort zone evaporates. To sustain your enthusiasm, connect your goals to making a difference in the life of someone you love. Make your own goals inspire others and appreciate how your loving self-care will likely keep you here on the planet longer for your loved ones. Significant, long-term motivation is an inside job.

Motivation is powerful medicine for the mind that can heal even the most limited beliefs in one's self. Its power comes from the fact that *you* have the choice/ability to create it and to allow it to move you to the highest success, happiness, and fulfillment. Where do you look for motivation—books, tapes, friends, family, seminars? All of these can offer motivation; just keep in mind that it is still you who holds the key to your own sustained motivation, and you can use it any and every time you desire to unleash it.

In coaching thousands of people over the last twenty years, we have found that the people who connected their goals, specifically weight-loss goals, to the work of total body and life transformation were the ones who experienced sustained inspiration, which carried them through to their successful outcome and desire. We are moved to make things happen and to do what is necessary—the work, sacrifice, diligence, and discipline—when we know the bigger *why* behind our movement.

Think of the *whys* you wrote down earlier. As you get more in touch and aligned with your intrinsic motivators, you become more committed to sharing your time and energy in only positive ways. In this moment, re-examine what intrinsically drives you, and get excited about your great big and compelling *why*. In these motivators lies the gold—all the fuel you will need on your journey. Allow motivation to come from your essential nature and sustain you for a lifetime.

When you are setting goals and creating intentions, consider what it is that you are looking for. Motivation is more sustainable when we come to the realization that we're not in this alone; everything we think, do, and say impacts those around us. This is one reason why the TEMT plan is so powerful: when we transform our own lives, we raise the ambitions of those around us, and that creates the space for everyone to come alive and thrive. Authentic happiness and peace of mind is shared and experienced together.

Think about a time when you wanted to achieve a certain goal—maybe a weight loss goal, or perhaps a financial or professional goal. There is a good chance that this goal involved others or affected those around you. Individuals rarely reach a goal when it is purely self-motivated. When you include in your goals the people who will also benefit through your discipline and efforts, you will be more likely to do whatever is necessary to realize it.

People who are change agents are intrinsically motivated: they always come from love! They attach the change they want to make to something bigger than themselves. When you know that your pursuits are not just about your own needs, you will not give up, sell out, or fail to do what needs to be done. The incentive is a deep knowing in your heart that keeps you moving forward and building resilience. This is how James was encouraged to change his unhealthy history and relationship with alcohol. This change inspired and opened him to pursuing a new circle of friends who lived healthier lives. He discovered his love for health and wellness, and it led him to becoming a doctor. Changing this one relationship supported him in transforming his life.

Who we hang out with the most tends to be who we become. Motivational speaker (and one of James's mentors) Jim Rohn famously said, "You are the average of the five people you spend the most time with." Because of this, we love the powerful practice of "peopling" our lives with people who inspire us. While there are exceptions to the rule, we believe in the law of averages and the idea that we must consciously place ourselves in environments that support our own growth and well-being. How does this work? It's really pretty instinctive.

Love More, Live Longer

Get connected and improve your chances of having a large 100th birthday celebration. When you have a tight and loving circle of friends enveloping your life, you will enjoy half the mortality rates as lonely people.[2] Stronger relationships also enhance overall survival rates. Women experiencing breast cancer have superior survival rates when they have ten or more close friends.[3] Even if you tend toward being more introverted, you can still expand your community—not by hoping to see it grow but by taking the initiative to serve others.

Spend the most time with people who raise you up, not bring you down. Read and watch things that teach and inspire. When you find yourself in a gossipy situation, excuse yourself. If you are hanging out with people who like to party every night and eat unhealthy food, it may be time to find a new tribe. If you live in a community of naysayers, start an optimist group to raise your vibration.

Courageous, committed change is a gateway to making life an amazing and inspiring experience of growth, love, and fulfillment. Intrinsic motivation and peopling our lives with encouraging individuals inspires us to discover our purpose—and then become a source of inspiration for others.

 Intrinsic Versus Extrinsic Motivation:
http://youtu.be/x6Tt1xOYgl0

. . . .

ACTION STEP
Write down one goal and reflect on *why* you are motivated to reach it.

My goal is: _____

My intrinsic motivation is: _____

. . . .

Your Personal Mission and Vision

When making changes, a personal mission statement clarifies your purpose and gives you a sense of direction. It defines who you are (or want to become) and how you want to live; it is your guiding light—your credo. Though it may take time to develop, as it requires thoughtful consideration, your mission statement is essential to your TEMT foundation.

One of the most important roles of a board of directors is to make sure an organization is staying true to its mission. We can do this same thing in our own lives by creating a personal mission statement and asking friends and family to be "the board" that holds us accountable.

• • • • • • • • • • • •

ACTION STEP

Create a space and time to think about and create your own personal mission statement. Focus on who and what you want to become. Keep it positive. Make it emotional. Infuse it with passion. Then read your mission statement aloud at least once a day.

Here is one that Dr. James wrote:

My mission is to serve the world with passion, integrity, purpose, courage, and love. Through leading-edge ideas, practical life strategies, and world-class service, I seek to encourage the healthy transformation of people and the planet.

And here are a few supportive prompts for your consideration:

My purpose is to express: _____

My mission is to become: _____

• • • • • • • • • • • •

Successful individuals and organzations have a vision. His Holiness the Dalai Lama's vision for a free Tibet is: "Future Tibet will be a peace-loving nation, adhering to the principle of *ahimsa* [nonviolence]. It will have a democratic system of government committed to preserving a clean, healthy, and beautiful environment. Tibet will be a completely demilitarized nation."[4] Successful organizations create a vision for their company, and churches have a vision for their congregation. It makes sense that successful individuals create a vision for their own life.

You my already have a vision for your life. Perhaps your vision involves your life as a mother or father, grandparent, head of a company, entrepreneur, global leader, famous actor, missionary for peace, Ironman triathlete, chef, or healer. No matter where you are in your current life or your current vision, you have the potential to make it even bigger and bolder. Your life's vision is similar to your mission, but it is more of an out-picturing of your aspirations for yourself and the world. Like your mission, your vision flows forth from your life purpose but applies to the greater whole. Your vision is a description of what you want your life to look life in order to achieve your purpose on the planet. Your vision has color, texture, and feeling; and it is most effectively accessed through the practice of meditation. The process of visioning (creating your visions) is a lot like becoming still and listening to your inner voice or your higher power—call it God, Allah, Buddha, Love, Krishna, the Universe—and allowing the vision to come.

Take some time to get clear about the vision for your life; listen for it, see it. Begin with thinking about what you really want to happen (aka magical thinking). Think about who and what inspires your vision. Your vision is what you want your life to look like in the near future. Write down your vision and read it daily, until you really embody the vision. Your vision is the moment-by-moment legacy that you can live every second of your day. If your mission is your road map, your vision is what your destination looks like.

· · · · · · · · · · ·

ACTION STEP

Have a vision of what you want to be, do, and have in your life. See it to be it. The mind loves to be visually fed. We are wired to picture virtually every thought we have. Visualizing the body, the experiences, the goals completed, and the vitality that you desire is powerful food for the mind. The more you visualize your life vision, the higher the likelihood that it will become your reality.

Visioning is slightly different than visualizing or visualization. Remember, visioning is the process of describing and visualizing what you want your life to look like in order to achieve your purpose on the planet. Visualization is a process that we can do at any given moment. It is a practice where we use our mind and our imagination to picture a desired state either in the present or the future. It is a technique we can use to help reduce stress and tension and increase relaxation. Your vision in this context is an affirmation of what you want your life to look like. It is "the big picture" invoked through deep thought and reflection, and sometimes visualization. Visualization is the act of imagining or picturing certain scenarios in any given moment. When we do this unconsciously, it's called daydreaming; when we do it with intention, it's called visualization.

When you use visualization practices, you stimulate the occipital lobe of the brain—the visual processing center. Visualization helps you see your desires in action and can be a strong source of inspiration. Set an intention, and schedule a time to visualize twice daily. Fill your mind with powerful images first thing in the morning and just before bed. Add this to your daily bookends, beginning and ending your day with the images of your desire, so your whole day is centered around building a path to the realization of your goals. Surround yourself with positive images that inspire, whether that be on your desk at work or on your refrigerator or altar. Let the images serve as a reminder of the powerful intentions you have set for yourself and your life's vision and mission.

• • • • • • • • • • • •

Exercise: Inspired Tools for Creating Your Life Vision

Before you begin the process of writing down the answers to some of the questions below, take time for meditation. Sit quietly and think about what your life would be like if you had the power to change it right here, right now. Focus on your gifts and talents. Ask yourself, *What do I need to know in this moment? What is it that I came here to do?* Remember, it is never too late to reinvent yourself. Here are other life areas where you may ask yourself questions:

My vision for my career:
What is my dream job?
How many hours do I work a day at this job?
What is my income?
Who do I work with?
How does my job make me feel?

My vision for family/relationships:
What are the qualities I desire in a partner?
What are the fun things we do together as a couple?
What are my qualities as a partner?
Do I see myself with children?
Who am I as a parent?
How do my friends describe me? (Remember this is the vision of who you are becoming.)

My vision for health and vitality:
What type of exercise do I do?
How many days a week do I exercise?
What do (and don't) I eat to stay healthy?
How do I feel physically and emotionally?
How do I support myself emotionally and spiritually?

My vision for my lifestyle:
Where is my ideal place for living?
What type of home do I live in?
How is it decorated?
How often do I take vacation?
Where do I love to travel?
How do I give back to the community through service?
How do I continue to improve my life through learning?

My vision for the planet:
What is my highest vision for the world?
How do I see individuals relating?
What do I wish to see now in the world—the most immediate changes?

From your answers, by choosing the ones that resonate the most, you can create a vision statement. This may be a sentence, a few sentences, or a paragraph. Write down your vision in first person, as if you are writing an autobiography. (You can do this as an individual exercise, with a small group of close friends, or as a family.) Then keep your vision statement somewhere you will look at and read it regularly.

Author Check-In

Debra's vision: I am committed to personal excellence, happiness, optimism, and spiritual growth. I am a positive role model for my daughters, who I love and support unconditionally. I compassionately serve those whose freedom has been restored, and I work tirelessly to help bring awareness and put an end to human trafficking and the devastating effects it has on millions of innocent lives. I am a trustworthy, loving, passionate, and supportive partner for my husband. I support my healthy mind and body with vigorous daily exercise, vital and organic whole foods, daily spiritual practice, and loving self-care. I live in a beautiful mountain community of moderate size with easy access to clean water, natural foods, and true friends. I am a nutrition and lifestyle medicine expert and leader in the field of women's hormonal health. I am a lover of animals, supporter of the less fortunate, and a loyal and committed friend to my close circle of friends.

2

THINK Confidence

Lack of confidence is largely due to SAD and our media addictions, be they Facebook, Twitter, the nightly news, newspapers, or tabloids. The media comes at us from many different avenues now, and it is constantly showing us how we are not good enough—at least that is how many of us take it in. It shows us that we need to look a certain way or own certain things to be a good person, and this creates a vicious cycle of making us feel small and insufficient. It also tells us the answer is outside ourselves. In reality, the first step to positive change is realizing just how amazing we already are and growing our confidence from there—so we truly know and embody the belief that we are capable of change, revealing the wonderful person we have inside us.

I Am Enough

You are now beginning the greatest work of your life: the work of spirited restoration and inspired self-awareness. Now is your time to step up and take your place in the life that you came here to create—if you choose to do the work. Times of darkness and perceived failure do not matter anymore. Be at peace with the knowledge that the work is lifelong, as it should be; it is your whole life's wellness we're offering. Let go of the quick-and-easy method, the deadlines, and the rush for immediate gratification—a mode of being that is not only unsustainable but also disappointing, and can easily erode your confidence. Only daily growth will allow for a successful journey.

We want to teach you how to successfully and sustainably create the life, body, and relationships that you desire and deserve using TEMT; TEMT is a way of life. It's about making choices every day and every moment that reflect the person you are here to be and become. You are already on the path of changing your habits and starting to create new ones, and there will be challenges on this road. You may slip up—whose life doesn't have these moments? While we encourage you to have self-discipline, we also encourage you, first and foremost, to remember self-compassion. We tend to hold on tightly to memories of tough times, our perceived screw-ups, and past disasters; and we tend to easily forget all the times we were amazing, smart, successful, and brave!

Somewhere in between adolescence and young adulthood, we adopt the majority of the habits and beliefs that will shape who we are and how we show up in the world. For some of us, this means that by the time we reach adulthood, we have taken on many less-than-healthy beliefs, habits, and ideas. We accept a bunch of untruths that society, family, environment, and the like have pushed on us; we drag around a less-than-awesome image of ourselves. This type of thinking makes us feel like we are chronically not enough, creating a negative cycle of limiting beliefs. And this chronic *not enoughness* has become widespread.

How can you successfully resurrect faith in yourself? Where are you right now in your self-love and self-awareness? Do you know that you are enough? Do you know that you have more to discover and to share?

With each and every move we make in the direction of our healing, the quest for serving and becoming our true selves creates more confidence and conviction. The fire gets stoked, and we want more. Our desire to show up and live the life that is ours becomes insatiable. We just need to work a bit harder to mine for our magic. Fortunately, we can get to it by simply leveraging the power of mindfulness and gratitude. Take the time to notice the good and the good will grow.

•   •   •   •   •   •   •   •   •   •   •   •

ACTION STEP

Reflect on your present life and all that is good. Notice the smaller (micro) daily joys along with the big-picture (macro) aspects, including family, accomplishments, and creative endeavors that you may have taken for granted. Focus on the good.

We tend to focus on the things in our lives that haven't gone well rather than the hundreds of things that have. In our busy and multitasking lifestyles, we can lose touch with our genius and all the greatness that we have achieved. You know the difference between when you're living your full potential and when you're slacking off. If you feel like you're not enough, it is time to take an inventory of life to figure out where that feeling is coming from. Check in with yourself. Are you on purpose—your life's purpose? Are you surrounding yourself with positive influences?

If you answer no to either or both of these questions, it doesn't mean that you aren't enough; it means that it is time to get back on track. Begin by surrounding yourself with individuals who support your mission and vision—individuals who inspire you to be your best self. Let go of what isn't working in your life and don't look back. Look ahead, and focus on your greatness.

•   •   •   •   •   •   •   •   •   •   •   •

Author Check-In

Debra's reflection: Chronic *not enoughness* has been a real source of pain for me. I never felt smart enough, pretty enough, thin enough, strong enough, funny enough, or worthy of positive praise or attention. I adopted these beliefs sometime in early childhood, in spite of receiving love and praise. I think this is common in children of divorced parents or alcoholics. "If only I were enough, they'd still be together"; "If I were more, they wouldn't drink." Even through counseling and support groups where I logically understood that I had nothing to do with anyone's drinking or marriage dissolving, it took (and continues to take) years of spiritual practice to arrive at a place where I know that I am enough. *The work I do is enough. My physical appearance is enough. My love for my family and friends is enough. My house is enough. My car is enough. My wardrobe is enough. My kindness is enough*, and so on!

It is still difficult for me to receive compliments; I have to remind myself daily that I am enough. And since I know this is true for me, I know it is also true for you. Let me reassure you: You are enough. You are worthy. You are whole.

Fire Your Critic and Hire Your Coach

How do you talk to yourself? Do you adore and unconditionally stand up for yourself; or do you talk to, judge, and treat yourself in such a way that if someone else were to treat you that way, you would never consider them your friend? Imagine having an inner dialogue with yourself that is unconditionally loving and supportive of your life's mission. Imagine you're having this dialogue with a coach who meets you first thing in the morning and encourages you to go after the day with passion and purpose. This coach knows your every dream and desire, and holds you to making them come true with conviction and unbridled enthusiasm.

Well, guess what? You already have this inner coach, and she can serve you as long as you listen to and follow her teaching!

There is a powerful parable about paying attention to the way we speak to ourselves:

An old Cherokee chief was teaching his grandson about life. "A fight is going on inside me," he said to the boy. "It is a terrible fight between two wolves. One is evil—he is anger, envy, sorrow, regret, greed, arrogance, self-pity, guilt, resentment, inferiority, lies, false pride, superiority, self-doubt, and ego. The other is good—he is joy, peace, love, hope, serenity, humility, kindness, benevolence, empathy, generosity, truth, compassion, and faith. This same fight is going on inside you—and inside every other person too." The grandson thought about it for a minute and then asked his grandfather, "Which wolf will win?"

The old chief simply replied, "The one you feed."

Who do you feed? Who gets your attention, and who do you listen to and follow—your inner coach or your inner critic? Most of us, especially those still living the SAD lifestyle, are fed information and media that, in turn, feeds the angry wolf. But you can change the game and transform every moment of your life, making it an epic affirmation of love and living. You can move from gossip and criticizing to awareness and love. Set the intention, and be bold in your conviction to challenge any limiting thoughts, outdated beliefs, or small thinking that you have dragged around for too long.

A Balanced Media Diet

The average American watches four hours of TV per day, which will stack up to taking nearly thirteen years of our lives. Psychologists say that the more you watch, the lower your self-esteem.[1] It is a "mean screen."

Consider how you might be using media for sustenance. How does your present media diet feed you? Do you feel satisfied after you watch the evening news? Does your morning-news fix energize you for the day? The mainstream media seldom inspires confidence and creativity, so it is important to use the media mindfully—if at all.

Watching the news can increase the risk of depression and anxiety.[2] Be conscious with what you place in your environment. The mind is permeable and can absorb almost anything it sees and hears.

When we think of going on a fast, we often think of food and the idea of going without. One of the empowering aspects of fasting from the news, reality shows, and so on is that we gain possibly dozens of hours each week that can be used to feed our mind, body, and spirit with much more nourishing "food." It takes courage and discipline to let go of the drama that is media, but wait until you see what happens when you tune in to your own personal greatness.

Switch the habit of flopping in front of the news each night by grabbing a friend, pet, or family member and taking a thirty-minute walk. Instead of opening the paper every morning to see how bad things are, choose to read a book or meditate and get yourself fired up for the day. You are in charge of the media that you allow into your life. If you are feeling full of bad news or simply feeling down, now is the time to turn off the TV and become more present in your life.

Notice that much of our thinking is limited, worn out, recycled, or even simply untrue. This type of thinking is a habit or reflex that we turn to unconsciously. You can shift your reactive thinking and change your inner dialogue paradigm by simply identifying and being mindful when you are in that SAD place.

•   •   •   •   •   •   •   •   •   •   •   •   •

ACTION STEP

When you are in a negative mindset, question it, call it out, refute it, and replace it with the truth of who you are. When you stand for your truth and follow it with an affirmative action, such as doing the right thing or following through on a good intention, you starve the critic and she eventually withers away. At the same time, your inner coach is being nourished and heard, and she steps up again and again, alive to the game of life. For example:

> Negative thought: I am too weak. I'll never be able to lose weight and eat healthy.
> Solution: I am building willpower daily, and my healthy choices are becoming a consistent part of my abundant life.

·   ·   ·   ·   ·   ·   ·   ·   ·   ·   ·   ·   ·

Author Check-In

Debra's personal example:
Negative thought: I am either too picky, not cool enough, or not interesting enough to attract new, like-minded friends into my life.
Solution: I am building courage and confidence; and attracting interesting, fun, and empowering friendships is becoming a consistent part of my life.

Now it's your turn.

Negative thought: I _____.

Solution: I am building _____, and

_____ is becoming a consistent part of my life.

Dr. James on Willpower:
http://youtu.be/sTSLPIcqlt8

Kick *But*

For many of us, the first step in creating a new experience and a new life is reducing how much we rely on our *but*. Do you use it for excuses? Does it keep you from moving forward in your life? It can be used in many creative ways to keep you living small and to perpetuate a mediocre life. Your *but* may be cloaked in the illusion of safety. It may be perceived as a good way of keeping things as they are, not making waves, and staying under the radar. It can be used as a way to avoid disappointment and avoid pain.

Your *but* may keep you from an amazing present and future: *I should exercise*, but . . . *I would like to change*, but . . . *I know that if I committed this time things would change*, but . . . But *what if I fail?* But *what happens if . . . ?* Your *but* keeps you from abundant living. Use it often enough, and it will keep you from achieving your big life goals—from having the experiences that will transform your life. A life of *buts* will absolutely keep you down, hold you back, and turn your life into a life of excuses, not only feeding your inner critic (the angry wolf) but also keeping you complacent.

How do you kick *but*? The first step is one we've already worked on: identify your bigger *why*. Decide *why* you need to overcome your history, and realize that holding on to *but* will only keep you from the life that you are here to live. See the life beyond your big *but*. Feel the energy and satisfaction of transcending your history; and know that the confidence and peace you deserve and desire will be created with each and every move you make to conquer *but*'s limitations and fully express your truth and purpose!

Pessimism vs. Optimism

Did you know that pessimism is related to higher levels of inflammation? A study performed at the Mayo Clinic over a thirty-year period showed that pessimists had a shorter life expectancy and an increase in the likelihood of developing Alzheimer's disease.[3] Researchers at the Harvard School of Public Health cited similar findings.[4]

Being an optimist is not a trait that you are lucky to be born with, and it is not made by having a lot of money or good looks. It's made the old fashioned way—by living it and building it!

One of the most common and, frankly, lame *buts* is "I would try to change this, *but* I got it from my family's bad genes, so my actions really won't matter." How we live—how we Think, Eat, and Move—has a powerful influence over our health and wellness. Our behaviors and actions are critical components in determining quality and length of life. We encourage you not to buy into the idea that your behavior is predetermined by your genes. Self-determination and the resolve to evolve are part of what makes us human. You hold the keys, and now it's time to put them in the ignition and take action.

•   •   •   •   •   •   •   •   •   •   •

ACTION STEP

A practice in kicking *but*:

1. Enlist the support of one or two friends or colleagues to support you in your mission and vision. If they hear you use *but* as an excuse to live small, ask them to give you a gentle nudge to remind you of your greatness.

2. Keep a journal nearby. Whenever you start to make an excuse for why you can't do something, write it down. Ask yourself: Is this really true? For example, if your quandary is, "I want to exercise, *but* I don't have enough time," we can help you see that's not true. For example, if you found time to write it down, you have time to exercise. If you have time to sit and watch an episode of *Cupcake Wars*, you have time to exercise. If you have time to peruse Facebook, you have time to exercise. It's all about priority, and when you make that priority exercise, you can always find the time.

3. Be courageous. Take your new attitude and refuse to make excuses public. If you saw the movie *Yes Man*, you may remember its premise: The main character, played by Jim Carrey, had to say yes to basically any and every opportunity that presented itself, no matter how outrageous. Of course this got him into some very interesting situations. It also kicked his *but* because he was no longer able to come up with excuses for not doing something. Channel your inner Yes Man or Yes Woman and you'll kick your own *but* out of the way.

• • • • • • • • • • • •

Every time you positively shift a thought and choose a new action, you will be reminded how good you really are. Witnessing your choice to be and express in an amazing way rather than an average one can become wonderfully addicting. Seeing your good is a practice of heightened awareness. And the brain is wired for efficiency, so any shift in thinking is a step toward overcoming a rut and rewiring your brain for the better.

 Dr. James on Positivity:
https://www.youtube.com/watch?v=NrDoQJQh0XI

Crafting Confidence

Confidence is rooted in knowing that you are enough, that your *why* is more powerful than your *but*, and that your inner coach can kick your inner critic's tail. Confidence is made and sustained through doing things consistently. Choosing one thing that you are going to work on is one of the most successful ways to boost confidence, make change happen, and be supported over the long term. Doing one thing well and owning it may be contradictory to our ego's desire to do and have it all, but the beauty in doing one thing well is that it allows for our mind to fully process, enjoy, and feel good about ourselves, creating a positive and lasting change. This is the TEMT mindset.

Author Check-In

Debra's reboot: One of the wackiest but most effective things I do when I feel like I am headed into a slump, or need a boost in creativity or confidence, is to find the nearest wall with clear floor space in front of it. I place my hands on the floor about six inches or so in front of the wall, and I kick up into a supported handstand against the wall. When I am in this position, the only thing I can focus on is my balance. I often try to come away from the wall with my feet and simply hold the handstand on my own. Sometimes I am successful; other times, not so much. When I am ready, I bring my legs down from the wall and come to my knees. I take a moment to find my center before I stand up. Once up, I shake out my arms, and I'm ready to dive right in to my next adventure.

One thing that sabotages confidence is multitasking. Multitasking is not good for our bodies or our brains. When we skip from task to task, the brain has to send signals to different areas of the body, which can cause stress on the immune system and create a tendency toward anxiety and low-grade depression. We do our best when we do one thing, complete it, enjoy the feeling of successful completion, and then move on to the next task. This is one way that we build confidence. When we allow ourselves to get caught up in keeping several balls in the air at one time, our minds suffer.

One way we experience success and feel positive about ourselves is by acknowledging the completion of a task or project. The mind and spirit need to feel the success of completing a task and, more specifically, doing one thing well. Begin today by choosing to do just one thing at a time. Focus on that one thing, and see it through to completion before moving on to the next task. Experiment with just washing the dishes; just driving your car; focusing on and listening to your spouse, child, or friend, and being there and nowhere else. Initially, this may be very uncomfortable. Your mind may want to go other places, your hands may fidget, and your body may feel antsy. This is a practice. Over time, you will gain greater control, greater mastery, and eventually deeper peace. This practice in living well will support you in making every relationship and every experience more meaningful. Your character and integrity will be sound and powerful—and your confidence will grow with every act done with awareness.

One key to growing self-confidence is to keep agreements with and commitments to yourself and others. This builds integrity, which is another confidence builder. Integrity is about choosing to show up, take action, and follow through on your good intentions. We create confidence by doing what we said we would do, regardless of whether or not we feel like it. Look around your life and notice what you have created by keeping agreements and following through. You are the witness to your life, and you know when you are being honest—in integrity—and when you are not.

Choose an area of your life, perhaps your health and well-being. There are certain practices that enable vitality to be realized in any area of your life, but they must be done with confidence and consistency. For example:

- Think: Spend five minutes in the morning and before bed writing down five things you are grateful for.
- Eat: Eat healthy and menu plan. (The TEMT Program at the back of this book can help make this easy!)
- Move: Block out time or times in your day for movement. If you only have fifteen minutes, make them count, and go for high-intensity intervals.

Confidence grows and diminishes in relationship to follow-through: it is all about doing what you know needs to be done, doing what you said you would do, and doing it daily. There is a lot of power in this simple practice, as it will allow you to find peace and power. It will afford you a life with clarity of purpose and the belief that you can create anything that you desire, because your experience of yourself has been one of showing up and doing what needs to be done.

For many, mastering the art of doing the daily fundamentals is not going to sound, feel, or appear fun or sexy. We get that. But there is a cool, sexy side effect of doing the daily good. As you commit and recommit to doing what needs to be done, your sense of confidence will increase. And confidence is sexy. Begin right now by just reading; do nothing else. How do you feel after accomplishing this singular goal for fifteen minutes or even an hour?

Confidence and a healthy self-esteem build the foundation for positive thinking. People your life with positive thinkers and people of great integrity. TEMT gives you the tools to create lasting confidence and the fortitude to grow your life from average to amazing. You are enough. You have the tools. There is no need to let your *but* get in the way of thriving.

Exercise: Confidence Check

Consider the following questions and activities, and write down your responses in your journal or notebook:

- List the top three accomplishments in your life that you are most proud of. What were the emotions you felt when you accomplished them?
- Who are the five people that you spend the most time with? How do you feel when you are around these people?
- Name at least three people that you would like to spend more time with.
- List the top three things that bring you the most joy in life.
- Now list the top three areas where you perceive you are lacking or limited in your life. On a scale of 1 to 10, rate each perceived area of lack in terms of how greatly it affects your life (with 10 being the most influential or limiting).
- List three action steps you could take today to relinquish that sense of lack or limitation. In other words, what could you do to bring that number closer to a 1 or 0?

Creating action steps and following through with them is a sure-fire way to build confidence. These questions and action steps may take you outside of your comfort zone, but they will increase your confidence even more. In answering these questions, trust that you have the potential to create the life of your dreams.

Author Check-In

Debra's debut: One morning, when our youngest daughter was quite young (under two years old), I had just turned on the TV to check the weather as I rode the exercise bike down in our basement. The bottom of the screen was flashing something like: "Auditions for *Rent* today at 2:00 PM, Denver Center for the Performing Arts." I had never seen *Rent* on stage, but I had heard great things about it, including the music. (I think I knew one song from the show at that time.) I had always thought of myself as a closet Broadway "wannabe," and in the moment I saw that TV ticker, there was something within me that said (shouted, actually), "It's now or never! You have to do this today or you never will!"

So I found someone to watch our daughter, and I tried to memorize a LeAnn Rimes song that I could sing at the audition.

Now, there are a few interesting things about this. First, if you've seen the show, it's not really aligned with LeAnn Rimes's music. And while I can carry a tune for the most part, I'm not someone who typically has the confidence to sing in front of others. Realistically, I'm just not that talented in the vocal department. But there I was, on a weekday that I happened to have off, driving to downtown Denver to audition. I was probably thirty at the time (trying out for a cast of twenty-somethings).

To make a long story short, I showed up, signed in ("Acting experience?" *Ummmm, doctor, mom, Tin Man in* The Wizard of Oz *in fifth grade . . .*), and waited my turn. I was definitely the oldest one there and my nerves nearly got the best of me, as I could hear every single note being belted out in the audition room by those who were called in before me. Finally, my turn came. To say I was a nervous wreck or even less than stellar would be kind, but they thanked me for my time, I thanked them in return, and off I went. Once I hit the parking lot, I was grinning ear-to-ear, tears streaming down my face. In that moment, I felt like what I had just done was the most uncomfortable personal experience I had ever had. Becoming a doctor and a mother seemed easy in comparison to that small blip of time, but the confidence I gained from doing something that really stretched every bit of me was off the charts—something I will never forget. And, no, I did not get a call back, but I did go on to see several performances of *Rent* and love that I will always feel a special connection to it.

3

THINK Power

Positive thinking, clarity, focus, patience, and confidence are created when the chemicals in our brain and bloodstream are balanced. How we think impacts every area of our life. So if our thinking is clouded by a chemical imbalance, deficiency, or excess of neurotransmitters or hormones, chances are we won't perform at our highest and best potential. In fact, we may feel depressed, insecure, distracted, cranky, sinister, or all of the above. TEMT gives you the tools to help build balanced brain chemistry so that you become literally wired for success.

Neurotransmitters and How to Use Them

Our thoughts and how we Think have everything to do with our brains and, more specifically, our brain chemistry. How we Eat and Move directly impacts our brain chemistry as well, which is why eating well and moving daily are essential components for clarity, positivity, calmness, creativity, and happiness. The human brain, a three-pound organ that sits suspended in a fluid cushion inside the skull, accounts for about

2 percent of your total body weight, but it burns 20 percent of your body's fuel.

The brain is the control center of the body and is made up of more than one hundred billion neurons. Each one of these neurons (nerve cells) can be connected by synapses to ten thousand other neurons. Messages travel from neuron to neuron with the aid of chemical communicators called neurotransmitters. When enough neurotransmitters build up in the synapse, the neuron fires, signaling other brain cells to fire. This communication ripple effect happens when you are trying to figure out a problem, answer a question, or muster up the conviction to push through a challenge; neurotransmitters are the chemicals that make all these things happen. These über-powerful brain chemicals ultimately determine how we perform and how we feel, but our lifestyle choices have a profound and direct relationship to how these chemicals perform on our behalf. Living the TEMT lifestyle will help you make the most of this powerful pharmacy in your head.

Neurotransmitters are capable of producing awesomeness—or they can allow us to feel awful. Pleasure, motivation, passion, calm, balance, and confidence are created here. Neurotransmitters can be built through positive lifestyle habits, including exercise and clean, healthy eating, or they can be compromised by SAD (Standard American Diet). Putting neurotransmitters to work on your behalf—keeping them in balance— will create a positive mindset worthy of inspiring the very best, making you feel great, while imbalances will negatively impact your mental and physical health.

The fuel you feed your body is used as building blocks for how you think; your levels of enthusiasm, confidence, and resilience; and your overall mindfulness and well-being. By engaging neurotransmitters every time you Think, Eat, and Move, you Thrive. We all have the ability to optimize the power and potential of the many dozens of neurotransmitters that support high performance, resilience, optimism, and vitality; but we will only touch on five—the ones we lovingly refer to as the varsity neurotransmitters that, in our opinion, lay the foundation for powerful living. These are dopamine; serotonin; norepinephrine; GABA (gamma-aminobutyric acid); and a lesser-known neurotransmitter, anandamide.

Dopamine (or what James likes to call the "morning mystic") bumps up your brilliance and sets the stage for a great day every day. It is partially responsible for regulating pleasure, mood, learning, and focus; and it supports morning motivation, alertness, confidence, sustained energy, memory, and commitment. Dopamine also regulates motor behavior; it is the pleasure-and-reward chemical. When the big D is happening in your brain, you are sure to rock your world with awesomeness. You can boost the dopamine levels in your brain with things like

- herbs such as ashwagandha, St. John's wort, American ginseng, Ginkgo biloba, green tea;
- coenzyme Q10; and
- foods like fish, kale, eggs, apples, berries, spirulina, nuts, beets, chicken, and bananas.

 Dopamine and Setting Your Day
http://www.youtube.com/watch?v=z6j4vqdg5Qw&list=PLDF2
6DC5254801299

Serotonin, what we call the "balance and contentment" chemical, is a major player in the regulation of mood, appetite, sex drive, the sleep-wake cycle, and overall mood balance. Serotonin also has a role in memory, temperature regulation, learning, and cardiovascular system function. An imbalance or deficiency of serotonin is one of the most common contributors to mood disorders. When serotonin levels are down, so is our mood; we are more likely to feel irritable, short tempered, and less then our best self. Serotonin is made and sustained through the conscious choices of foods and movement, and mindfully managing stress by cultivating and demonstrating empowering habits of loving self-care.

Hormones and estrogen levels can affect serotonin levels, which may explain why some women have premenstrual and menopausal mood complaints. Some of the best ways to boost serotonin levels in our brain include

- eating healthy fats, especially omega-3 fatty acids from fish, nuts, and seeds;
- combining healthy complex carbohydrates with lean protein;
- exercising every day;
- having protein at each meal;
- eliminating sugary carbs, and eating whole grains and lots of dark-green leafy veggies;
- getting plenty of sleep (aim for eight hours per night, and try to get to bed before 10:00 PM);
- avoiding caffeine, alcohol, tobacco, and sugar; and
- surrounding yourself with people who love you, and hugging them often.

Become a Great Sleeper

Great sleepers are happier; more productive; and better at managing their weight, reducing the amount of calories they eat daily, and choosing better food. Great sleepers are happier, sexier, and stronger compared to poor sleepers. Unfortunately, most of us do not get enough quality sleep, and this lack of sleep increases our risk for many life-threatening lifestyle diseases. One of the fastest-growing classes of prescription drugs is for insomnia and sleep challenges.

Here are our top six strategies and supplements for great sleep:

1. Five-minute hot shower followed by a twenty-second cold blast

2. Melatonin (3 milligrams thirty minutes prior to laying down)
3. Relaxing yoga
4. Passionflower (herb)
5. Chamomile tea, Holy basil tea, or valerian root
6. No evening news/media, computer work, etc. before bed

Norepinephrine is the learning chemical. Chemically similar to dopamine, norepinephrine has a dual role as a neurotransmitter and a hormone. It helps support concentration, mood, and the formation of new brain cells. This key player is a major influence in decreasing brain inflammation and is the brain chemical most affected in Alzheimer's disease. Norepinephrine levels tend to be low when people suffer from depression or ADHD (attention deficit/hyperactivity disorder). To naturally increase norepinephrine in your brain,

- eat protein at each meal;
- get plenty of exercise;
- drink green tea; and
- eat bananas and dark-green leafy veggies.

Gamma-aminobutyric acid (GABA) is the neurotransmitter that helps us feel at ease and relaxed; it is the main inhibitory (calming) neurotransmitter in the brain. GABA receptors are stimulated by a glass of wine at the end of a harried day, for example, enabling relaxation and calm. Many sedatives enhance the effects of GABA too, but you can boost your GABA levels naturally by

- eating cherry tomatoes and shrimp;
- drinking oolong tea; and

• drinking kefir (Kefir is sometimes described as drinkable yogurt—it is a fermented product, usually made from cow's or goat's milk, but also coconut milk and even water. Kefir contains active live cultures [probiotics], B vitamins, calcium, and protein, and has a tart and sour taste. It has a thinner consistency than yogurt.)

Anandamide is a lesser-known neurotransmitter that offers pain relief and has a similar effect to that of marijuana. The name itself originates from the Sanskrit word *ananda*, which means "bliss." Thus anandamide has come to be known as the bliss molecule, helping us feel calmer, more centered, and clearer—a peaceful way to set the tone for evening bliss and restful sleep. Anandamide plays a role in the generation of motivation and pleasure, and is important for immune function. Research is still forthcoming in terms of ways to boost anandamide, though the EPA (eicosapentaenoic acid)/DHA (docosahexaenoic acid) from fish oils seem to be one of the best ways. Anandamide is also induced through exercise, particularly running.

The Hormone Connection

Neurotransmitters work together with another important family of chemicals called hormones. Whereas neurotransmitters act locally at the synapse, hormones travel through the bloodstream and act as messengers between cells. When neurotransmitters and hormones work together efficiently, our minds and bodies are at their best. Hormones affect circadian rhythms (our sleep-wake cycle), mood, metabolism, reproduction, menopause, hunger cravings, and arousal; they prepare the body for fight or flight and more. Hormones make things happen. We want to discuss just a few of them here.

Cortisol is our primary stress hormone. Cortisol levels are generally increased with chronic stress, poor sleep, excess caffeine intake, excessive exercise, and calorie restriction. Chronically elevated cortisol levels have been linked to weight gain, insulin resistance, type 2 diabetes, high blood pressure, depressed immune system, and decreased libido. In fact, high cortisol levels can affect all of our sex hormones: testosterone, estrogen, progesterone, and dehydroepiandrosterone (DHEA). Cortisol levels can also plunge as a result of chronic stress, leaving us feeling tired, burned out, and susceptible to illness, low blood pressure, and increased sensitivity to environmental stress and allergies.

DHEA serves as a precursor hormone for female and male sex hormones. DHEA is produced primarily in the adrenal glands (aka the stress glands), and surprise! Cortisol is produced in the adrenal glands too. The production of cortisol and DHEA can become imbalanced when we are under stress; and when DHEA is out of balance, the other sex hormones can become imbalanced as well. This can affect libido, performance, fertility, mood, and metabolism.

Allowing stress and cortisol to go unchecked will eventually take you down. Being in a chronic alarmed state leads to exhaustion; and lower levels of testosterone steal muscle, leading to lower levels of naturally occurring growth hormone (GH). Men who carry extra weight are at risk for lower levels of testosterone—and with that, their sexual performance may be less than stellar. They may be less likely to produce healthy sperm and sperm counts as well.

Growth hormone (GH) is an important part of healthy aging. GH levels are expected to decrease after thirty, forty, fifty years on the planet, but how well and strong you age is truly up to you—how you choose to allow it to unfold. You don't have to settle for anything less than feeling great! GH not only serves your physique but it also serves your brain, your mind, all your tissues, and your mood. Get excited for the possibility that your best and most awesome living is now and in the future!

You can naturally raise GH in the body through

- high-intensity interval training (HIIT);
- getting adequate sleep (at least eight hours a night); and

- eating a balanced diet with plenty of lean protein, while cutting out excess sugar (whey protein provides an easy way to do this, plus it contains the amino acid glutamine, which may boost GH levels).

Express Your Best

We've learned how neurotransmitters and hormones influence how we feel and perform, and we know that our environment—who and what surrounds us—also impacts our behavior. Mirror neurons are powerful brain cells whose job description is "copy others." Mirror neurons are a subset of motor neurons, which fire with physical action. One of the interesting things about mirror neurons is that they fire when observing someone else perform an action. If you witness someone slam their finger in a door, you flinch and say, "Ooh, ow!" We are wired to relate, to feel, and to want to follow what we see going on in front of us. Think of them as your empathy neurons.

A simple way to understand mirror neurons is to think about what happens when you see someone yawn. How do you respond? Most often you yawn. Consider this: You are feeling strong, energized, and optimistic. You are crushing your day and feeling high on life. Then you come in contact with a group of people who are having a bummer of a day. Their energy is way down, their body language stooped and withdrawn. Suddenly, you notice that you are starting to feel their collective bummer—you sort of take it on. Emotions are powerful, and they are contagious. You can catch others' emotions in the same way that you can spread yours. Mirror neurons are basically copycat cells in our brains that feel, sense, and live to follow what is going on around us. This mirroring happens automatically and subconsciously.

Mirror neurons allow us to empathize and communicate through facial expressions, and this works both ways. When you are expressing your best, it translates to others. Choose what you keep around you wisely. When you act with love, you eat well; move with gratitude; shine bright; and emote good, kind, and loving energy that others watch and copy. What a powerful and motivating responsibility!

People your life well. Remember that idea of being the average of the five people you hang out with most? Keep this in mind as you go about your life. You want to be around others who are positive just as much as you want to be a positive influence for others. If your closest friends or family members are constant complainers, pessimists, criticizers, or are just plain mean, it's time to move on and spend less time around them. Surround yourself with people and places that reflect your vision for your life.

 Dr. James on Mirror Neurons:
http://youtu.be/r92OZqyRx4A

Be It to See It or See It to Be It

When we surround ourselves with the people and places that reflect more of who we want to be, we begin to live the vision for our lives. We begin to say and do the things that people we admire say and do. You've probably heard the expression, "see it to believe it" or "see it to be it." Well, this can go both ways. We have to *be* the person we want to see show up in the world, but we can also *see* the person we want to be through visualization and using affirmations to help us *be* it.

Our brains are very teachable. When we set our minds to a certain goal and use visualizations and affirmations to work toward it, we are basically directing the frontal lobe of our brain, which serves as our body's commander in chief and makes all our decisions. In essence, we are instructing our brain through imagery to get on board with an idea and make it real. We see it to be it.

Coming at it from another angle, when we act *as if*, our actions and attitudes are more likely to manifest in real time. This is all about rehearsing the actions of the person you desire to be. When you demonstrate the actions of a successful person (even if you feel you are simply playing the part), you send a strong and direct message to your subconscious mind to find and create the experiences that enable your desired outcome to be realized. *Be it to see it* is the concept of training your brain to activate your body and mind to be the person you wish to be. A habit becomes a ritual through practice. The more our brains experience a certain behavior, the more likely it becomes a habit.

• • • • • • • • • • • • •

ACTION STEP

Pick the type of person you wish to be. For example: a morning person who gets up at 5:00 AM to meditate and exercise. The first several mornings will likely be a stretch for you emotionally and neurologically because the behavior is brand new, and there is a new neurological framework to develop. But your brain will neurologically fire, and over time, several days to weeks, begin to wire a new neurological pathway each time you practice being this morning person who is up at 5:00 AM, meditates, and exercises. The habit is built on systematically building strong neurological pathways by practicing being the person.

You have this power. Now you need to choose who to be and then act to see.

• • • • • • • • • • • • •

So how do you put these powerful practices into action? You simply do the work. Leverage visualization, affirmation, and your *why* by beginning to see the desired outcome. Trust that your brain is going to follow through on the order. From here, you need to practice being the person who you desire to see.

Get excited about using the brain for what it does best. It *imagines*. When you choose to dedicate time each day to visualize (to see what you wish to be) and to act as if (to be what you wish to see), you are quite literally training your brain to become its best and most powerful expression. Think of your brain like a muscle: it gets stronger with use. When our brains do not grow, our lives do not grow. You have the source of power, greater purpose, and success right between your ears; your "exercise" is your imagination. Give your brain a workout every day and you will build a fulfilling life of your dreams and desires.

· · · · · · · · · · · · ·

ACTION STEP
Rehearse the actions of the person you desire to become. Experience the feeling of being and seeing your highest and best self. If you are modeling someone else, see with their eyes the things and people they are seeing. Use all of your senses to truly embody your ideal you. Set the intention to look for ways and opportunities to embody this vision.

This exercise of acting *as if* is an opportunity to play and become intimate with your true self. It's all about stepping into the person of your dreams because he/she is the person that you truly are. Get used to this person because you'll be this person for a long time!

· · · · · · · · · · · · ·

Life as Meditation

One of the greatest rituals we have done for over twenty years is meditation. Meditation is one of the best ways (if not *the* best way) to help improve the way we think—about everything! As such, meditation is one of the core thinking practices of the TEMT Program. The Tibetan word for *meditation* is *gom*, and its literal translation is "to become familiar with one's self." It refers to training the mind for the positive. Creating a habit of meditation enables you to become honestly familiar with yourself; you come to terms with your current self and catch a glimpse of your possible self.

Dr. Jon Kabat-Zinn is the founding director and professor of medicine emeritus at the Center for Mindfulness in Medicine, Health Care, and Society at the University of Massachusetts Medical School. He teaches mindfulness meditation all over the world, defining mindfulness as "the awareness that arises by paying attention, on purpose, in the present moment, and nonjudgmentally."[1] The more time we can spend in this experience and this awareness, the healthier our attitudes and the healthier our brains. Mindfulness meditation may reduce loneliness[2]; it boosts concentration and strengthens immunity[3]; it decreases stress and promotes relaxation[4]; and it improves resiliency and equanimity (the ability to regain true self and balance).[5]

Mindfulness meditation is showing up in schools, corporate offices, professional sports teams, and operating rooms. It is a way of mentally focusing on being in the present moment; and it has even proven to be an effective tool in helping people with cognitive and behavioral issues after traumatic brain injury.[6] Meditation of all kinds, from chanting to visualization, reduces stress and promotes balance in the body.[7]

Sitting quietly for fifteen to thirty minutes a day can change your life. It creates a sense of centeredness, compassion, and clarity that supports a creative and balanced life. But if you are someone who believes you just can't sit still for that long, then begin with just two minutes.

• • • • • • • • • • • •

ACTION STEP

Find a quiet spot, close your eyes, and focus on your breathing—slow, deep inhalations and exhalations. Breathe in the thought of love or joy or peace, and exhale out worry, stress, and fear. Use your quiet sitting time to see yourself through eyes of love and compassion. Acknowledge the self that you no longer wish to be—the one who may settle for less than the best because of fear of or resistance to change. Thank the self for the learning experience, then consciously decide to change course to get back on purpose and intention.

. . . .

After you begin to meditate, you will hopefully start to feel some type of shift in your thoughts; and after a few times of practice, your mind may become more still. The old stressed or anxious you will begin to fade as your new, more confident self grows stronger. In essence, you are unplugging and unwiring from an old way of living and rewiring to energize a new you.

Think you don't have time to meditate? His Holiness the Dalai Lama begins and ends his days with two hours of prayer and meditation. He has said that on especially busy days, he will meditate even longer. If you have time for *Real Housewives of Anywhere*, you can certainly find time for meditation.

Author Check-In

James's meditation routine: I began meditating in earnest when I was in my midtwenties as part of a daily practice encouraged at the intentional community where I lived. I found meditation to be challenging at first, as creative types like me sometimes find it difficult to sit still and just be. In the last thirty years, I have participated in thirty-day silent meditation retreats as well as ten-day mindfulness retreats; and today, I am doing the work of sitting every morning before I jump into the busyness that is my life. Meditation has served me well on so many levels.

Before you decide whether or not you can or would meditate because you have a religious idea about it that does not fit, or you have a vision of being coerced into some kind of yoga pose that gives you cramps just thinking about it, let go of all of that; that's just another *but* getting in the way. Consider this daily practice a time-out for body and mind—an opportunity to let the busyness of your brain and life pause. One of the greatest benefits that meditation offers is the power of remembering who you are at your core. It connects you to your source and the truth of who you are beyond all the stuff that you tend to be identified with. Meditation is an elixir for your entire life; it's a blessing that will feed and support you in creating the experiences you desire, the resilience needed to overcome challenges, and the clarity and energy to express your highest self. It will help you Thrive!

Exercise: Simply Breathing

While certain disciplines have specific instructions, there are no real rules when it comes to meditating (though some may disagree); you can get started by simply sitting quietly. You can meditate sitting, standing, lying down (though it's not recommended since it's so easy to fall asleep), or walking.

Find a place where you can resist being distracted or interrupted. Begin by slowing down your breathing, inhaling and exhaling at a reduced pace; do not hold your breath. Do not hyperventilate either. Simply slow down, bringing your breathing down into your diaphragm. If you need a frame of reference, inhale slowly for four seconds and exhale for six seconds. You may find it helpful to recite a phrase or chant while you breathe.

See this practice as a non-negotiable part of your day, and schedule it as though it is your most important meeting. This practice offers the critical experience of aligning your choices and actions with your truth and purpose.

4

THINK Happy

Why did you pick up this book? Most likely, it was because you'd like to change something in your life. And whether that means thinking more effectively, eating more healthfully, or moving more often, these changes are all in service to one thing: your happiness. Being happy will help you thrive on a number of levels, not the least of which is helping your brain achieve its highest function.

The Happiness Factor

We have been studying happiness and what makes people happy for many years now, through research and our work with clients and patients. Personal health is one of the greatest determinants to happiness, and we believe authentic happiness serves to create a beautiful life. Happy people aren't just healthier, they live longer.[1]

If you were to ask the majority of people—from any culture, age, and socioeconomic background—what they want most in this lifetime, chances are they would say true happiness. But what does this really mean? What is true happiness? Is happiness the mere absence of sadness? Is it inner peace? Is it wealth? Health? Balance? Attaining a certain goal?

The truth is, happiness is difficult to quantify and define in a strict sense. In psychology, happiness is attributed to positive emotions such as optimism, contentment, self-esteem, and serenity. Happiness connotes a state of pleasure and satisfaction. It is a state that many Americans are struggling to attain and willing to pay big bucks and go to extreme lengths to achieve.

Happiness Is Contagious

Happiness is both self-serving and a selfless act of love. And happiness is contagious. Dr. Martin Seligman is regarded as the father of the modern positive psychology movement. He has researched positivity, optimism, and happiness for decades, and his findings are inspiring and awesome! There are many ways to get your smile on. His work is all about identifying what makes you happy, which Seligman refers to as finding your "signature strength" (SS)—the thing that you love to do.[2]

Give yourself permission to pursue your SS often. Ideally, your signature strength is something that stretches you, pushes your edges, and makes you grow. Doing what you love is an empowering process of opening your heart and giving yourself the gift of what you love. Happiness is a state of living and being that is yours to create, to share, and to openly ask for more of.

In 2010, Americans spent more than $16 billion on antipsychotic medication, $11 billion on antidepressants, and $7 billion on drugs to treat ADHD.[3] While medication is truly a lifesaver for many, too many of us turn to medication as the answer to our happiness or lack thereof; we believe we'll find happiness in a bottle rather than by looking within and changing our lifestyle. We may compare ourselves to people who are happy and think that medication will give us that same level of happiness. We attach conditions to our happiness. For example, we're happy on Fridays since it's the end of our workweek, or we're happy when a certain person does something just the way we expected, or we're happy after a certain situation goes right. When things happen just the way we want them to, we assume we will finally be happy. But come Monday, forget it; it's Monday after all, the beginning of the workweek, of school, of being home alone. What if, instead of the Monday blues, we put on our Monday shoes and went for a run? That action alone would boost your spirits more than you may expect.

In Bhutan, a nation landlocked between India and China in the Himalayas, happiness is more important than the Gross National Product (GNP)—so much so that in 1972, the fourth King of Bhutan, His Majesty Jigme Singye Wangchuck, declared Gross National Happiness (GNH) to be more important than GNP. From that time forward, the national policy and development of Bhutan were oriented around GNH.[4] This philosophy, combined with knowing that the entire country is cheering you on, could certainly help bring a person out of a funk, wouldn't you agree?

For individuals with severe depression, medication may provide the necessary relief. For some, a daily exercise routine can help them emerge from a rut. Removing junk food from our diet and replacing it with whole foods, fresh fruits and vegetables, and clean proteins can help us all feel better in general.

We've thrown around terms like *authentic happiness* and *true happiness*, but we'd like to introduce another: *irrevocable happiness*—happiness that is unconditional; happiness that does not depend on anything going on outside of us. It is the kind of happiness that is always within us and cannot be taken away. When we clearly define what brings us joy no matter what the outside circumstances, we can always find a reason to smile. And this may serve as a jump start to taking the steps for change.

As naturopathic doctors, we have counseled many patients who have come in seeking alternatives to antidepressant medications. In addition to talking through therapy options, an exercise program, and healthy eating guidelines (similar to those outlined in our TEMT Program), there are natural therapeutic agents that support a more positive chemistry and greater overall happiness.

Here are some other happiness boosters: Get outdoors and into the natural sunlight. Sunlight stimulates the pineal gland, a small endocrine gland in the brain that produces certain neurotransmitters and the hormone melatonin, both of which greatly impact our mood. Sit by open windows and replace your light bulbs with full spectrum bulbs. Sunlight also stimulates the production of vitamin D, which many people need more of. Vitamin D deficiency has been linked to mood disorders and declining cognitive function,[5] so consider having your primary care doctor measure the vitamin D levels in your blood.

Maintaining a journal of emotions (and circumstances surrounding them) and progress along your TEMT journey can help to identify areas in need of attention. We recommend keeping a gratitude journal as well, where you record at least one thing that you are grateful for each day. This is a great way to keep looking at the bright side of things.

Natural Antidepressants

St. John's wort still tops the list as one of the most researched natural medicines for mild to moderate depressive mood disorders. As with any supplement or medication, it is best to consult your primary care doctor prior to self-medicating, no matter how minor you may feel your condition is. St. John's wort is a plant medicine that has been used for centuries for mood-related disorders, including mild to moderate depression and anxiety. The suggested dose of a standardized extract is 450 to 900 milligrams twice daily.

Low levels of S-adenosyl methionine (aka SAMe), produced in the body from the amino acid methionine, have been found in people with depression. SAMe has long been used by doctors in Europe to treat depression and is catching on in America. Research has shown that SAMe may be as effective as some pre-scriptive medications (tricyclic antidepressants) used to treat depression.[6] It is recommended that SAMe be taken in conjunction with a B-complex supplement (including folic acid and vitamin B12, which are needed to make SAMe) to avoid buildup of homo-cysteine, an amino acid that forms when SAMe breaks down in the body. A recommended dose of SAMe is 400 milligrams two to three times daily; and be forewarned, SAMe can be pricey.

High antioxidant foods like fresh berries, green tea, prunes, beans, and legumes help keep the body and mind healthy and happy. And complex carbohydrates in the form of whole grains, sweet potatoes, fresh fruits and vegetables, nuts and seeds, in addi-tion to wild fish, lean meat, and organic dairy products contribute to the building blocks for health and happiness.

Trust in yourself and maintain the attitude of an optimist. Know that it is okay to surrender to emotions other than happiness. True happiness is a way of being in the world; it is a core value. You can be a happy per-son even when life hands you sadness or grief, as long as you remember the irrevocable happiness that dwells inside of you.

Dr. James on Happiness
http://www.youtube.com/watch?v=NgNpG9A1cy-Q&list=PLDF26DC5254801299

• • • • • • • • • • • • •

ACTION STEP

Every night for the next ten nights, before you go to sleep, write down three things that you accomplished during the day. How did these things make you feel?

Challenge yourself to get outside daily. Enjoy the early morning or late afternoon rays of sunlight for just fifteen minutes before 10:00 AM or after 4:00 PM.

· · · · · · · · · · ·

Laugh to a Longer Life

We have a family ritual that on most evenings, we make time to laugh together. We love to get our happy on after a long and stressful day. After dinnertime, we'll put on some good, fun music during cleanup and dance together for at least one full song. At that time, James usually breaks out his conga drum skills (or lack thereof), and that, in and of itself, is fodder for extreme laughter. Our hearts and souls love it! We find especially good laughter material with our daughters and pets. Both of our girls inherited a keen sense of humor and wit and share the gift of seeing the sunny side of life. They are silly and bring a sense of lightness into the house so that we rarely take ourselves too seriously. Our pets are just funny, period. We have a pug who strikes the best poses, always with tongue out; and a basset hound who gets into mischief and loves to exercise his vocal talents. We find humor and lightness in ourselves as well, in our mistakes and missteps.

So, what makes you laugh or keeps you from laughing? Why should you laugh more often? Laughter helps us lighten up. Being rigid makes you appear old and inflexible, and it does the same to your heart and mind; it makes you less approachable. But laughter benefits your mind. When we see images or sights that are humorous, we tend to remember them better. Stretch your mind and memory by putting yourself in the midst of fun.

Robust belly laughter releases endorphins and reduces the stress hormone cortisol.[7] As we talked about in the last chapter, too much stress and cortisol can add weight around the midsection and lead to inflammatory challenges. Reducing cortisol and epinephrine with laughter may also help keep your heart healthy, as these two hormones play a role in heart disease and can weaken the immune system.[8] Simply anticipating laughter can increase growth hormone (GH) and beta-endorphins, boosting immunity and decreasing depression.[9]

Laughter even improves quality of life and resiliency in breast cancer survivors.[10] Our bodies fight off cancer better when we increase the activity of natural killer (NK) cells and antibodies. Laughter not only increases NK cells[11] but boosts endorphins, and with this boost, you see a decrease in pain and improved quality of life.[12] The blessing of laughter is real and far-reaching: it raises both our physiology and our psychology.

Laughter may be contagious too (remember those mirror neurons), offering similar benefits to anyone within earshot. So, develop the discipline (yes, discipline) of daily laughter. And if you can't always find the laughter, a simple smile can do the trick in lightening your mood and the mood of those around you. The gift of a smile is heart lifting and affirming—good medicine given or received.

• • • • • • • • • • • •

ACTION STEP

Spend at least fifteen minutes daily on frivolous laughter. If you are someone who takes life too seriously, you may want to get a few suggestions from your "funnier" friends. There are always funny pet videos online, funny movies, and friends who can deliver a great joke.

• • • • • • • • • • • •

Moving from Me to We

Researchers at Harvard Medical School studied the happiness of nearly five thousand individuals over a period of twenty years, and they found that when an individual becomes happy, the *network effect* can be measured up to three degrees. *Network effect* is a business term that describes the impact that one user of a product or service has on other people's value of the product. In our example of network effect, we are referring to the idea that one person's happiness can trigger a chain reaction that benefits immediate friends as well as their friends' friends, and their friends' friends' friends. And the effect lasts up to one year.[13]

People are happier, healthier, and far more effective in community.[14] Community may look like a close-knit neighborhood, spiritual congregation, book club, tennis team, or retirement community. When we involve ourselves in community, we work for the greater good of the group. An example of a close-knit neighborhood: we share meals; we watch each others' pets when someone goes out of town, we look out for each others' children and the elders of the neighborhood; we help keep things clean by picking up trash or planting trees; we know each others' birthdays and get together as a neighborhood at least a few times a year. Making this move from "me" to "we" can help you reach your goals of happiness, provided that your goals are also in alignment with the bigger picture of *we* or *us*. It is a move from selfish to selfless.

One of our spiritual mentors is Dr. Michael Bernard Beckwith. He embodies and inspires others to be a "beneficial presence" in the world. This means choosing to show up big, beautiful, and brilliant for the world to see. When you choose to be a beneficial presence, those who witness your actions and behavior benefit on many levels; and when people observe or experience your kindness and service, their levels of serotonin (the happiness hormone) can increase. This makes us wildly inspired and beckons us to put our creative, kind hearts in action. We've experienced this with kind neighbors who have plowed our driveway without us asking. We have seen this when we have shared food or healthy treats with friends and neighbors and then observed how much it makes their day, or helps them to take their healthy habits to a new level and share with others. As we have shined our lights within our communities, we have received the blessing of so much in return. It's this act of selfless service and social activism that leads us to thriving in life.

 Moving From Me to We
http://www.youtube.com/watch?v=oHtrPm-WIDOg&list=PLDF26DC5254801299

• • • • • • • • • • • •

ACTION STEP

Keep track of how many times you use the words "I," "me," or "mine" during the day.

Aim to reduce this usage by 25 percent during the next week and incorporate more "we," "us," and "our" into your vocabulary.

Do something today that gets you involved at a community level, such as volunteer, help a friend or neighbor in need, or attend a workshop.

• • • • • • • • • • • •

Gratitude is the Gift that Keeps On Giving

Dr. Robert Emmons is an expert in the science and power of gratitude. His research brings credibility to why we should all add more gratitude to our lives, showing that a conscious focus on blessings may have physical, emotional, spiritual, and interpersonal benefits. In one experiment, students who kept gratitude journals on a weekly basis were more likely to engage in regular exercise, reported fewer physical complaints, felt better about their lives as a whole, and were more optimistic about the upcoming week compared to those who recorded hassles or neutral life events.[15] In other research, Dr. Emmons and colleagues enrolled adults with neuromuscular disease and had them participate in a twenty-one-day gratitude study. Compared to a control group of people who did not write down things they were grateful for, those who participated in gratitude journaling reported better moods, more energy, more optimism, a deeper sense of connection with others, and greater quality and duration of sleep.[16]

In his book *Thanks!: How Practicing Gratitude Can Make You Happier*, Dr. Emmons writes about the "law of emotional contagion." He explains how individuals are "susceptible to 'catching' other people's emotions."[17] This isn't necessarily an original idea. Charles Darwin, Carl Jung, and other theorists noted that emotions were contagious as early as the late nineteenth century. Our emotions are influenced by the emotions of others and vice versa. This works in the positive and the negative sense of emotional contagion, which ties us back to the idea of peopling our lives with positive people who lift us up, not bring us down. The bottom line is that we take on the moods and attitudes of those around us; and at the same time, we are partially responsible for creating the moods of others.

Be the source of positive vibes. You have a choice every moment to express your appreciation for your life and all its gifts, from being able to breathe a deep breath to witnessing a child laugh to holding the hand of someone you love.

Optimistic Illusion

According to the National Institutes of Health "moderate optimistic illusion is essential to maintain motivation and good mental health."[18] Basically, you need to see yourself and the world through the lens of positivity. With that outlook, you will enjoy greater well-being than those looking at life through the eyes of pessimism.

Think about how you navigate your day when you are feeling optimistic. When you show up for your life with an optimistic mindset, it seems as though the entire Universe is rooting for your success and positive experience. Optimists and extroverts experience greater longevity compared to pessimists![19] Optimism may lead to improvement in cardiovascular outcomes in people with diagnosed cardiovascular disease.[20] Optimism may be the long-sought Fountain of Youth.

We believe that keeping a gratitude journal and making daily lists of things that you are grateful for are two of the most effective and meaningful ways to make progress toward important personal goals (whether they be related to health, academics, or your professional life). Children who practice "grateful thinking" have more positive attitudes toward school, their families, and themselves.[21] And you can grow gratitude simply by serving others.

When you are truly grateful, you place less emphasis on comparing yourself to friends, family, coworkers, neighbors, and celebrities. Having an attitude of gratitude helps to dispel depression, lower stress, and create a feeling of physical, emotional, and spiritual positivity. An attitude of gratitude lowers stress hormones like cortisol and increases DHEA.[22] The beauty in being grateful is knowing in your heart that gratitude gives back 100 percent.

Gratitude can serve to elevate your thinking and your motivation to achieve goals around self-care. Being grateful makes these things more likely to be realized, as it enhances our commitment and willingness to want to follow through and do what needs to be done. Gratitude acts as fuel for our *why* commitments, bringing extra firepower to sustain the journey. Be genuine, open your heart, and allow the gratitude to flow.

Dedicate yourself to a bedtime ritual: gratitude journaling. A five-minute session with your heart open and pencil in hand can help you to achieve many of the milestones of wellness you may have set for yourself.

Being grateful is a choice. It is all about how you look at the world and your desire to see the good—no matter how small—and celebrate it. And expressing your gratitude not only serves you in living your best life but it may also be a force that shifts and uplifts those in your midst. When it comes to the happiness factor and being authentically happy, gratitude is an essential part of the plan.

. . . .

ACTION STEP

What can you do right now that will grow your gratitude and happiness?

- Practice gratitude and kindness.
- Demonstrate your special gifts and talents.
- Have meaningful goals that stretch you and make you wonderfully uncomfortable.
- Practice a TEMT lifestyle.
- Be a student of life.
- Avoid comparisons.

. . . .

Whether you call it your job, your hobby, or your spiritual path, happiness is your birthright. You have the power to show up every moment of your life and build your happiness. The work is the process; the outcome is happiness. In fact, the overall experience will make you happier, and the daily actions that build this happiness will be contagious and inspiring to others. The more you put out the happy vibes, the happier you—and everyone around you—will ultimately be.

The Power of Gratitude
http://www.youtube.com/watch?v=9R8RfV-ghUO8&list=PLDF26DC5254801299

Exercise: Get Your Happy On

- Keep a gratitude journal. You don't even have to write every day; three to five times a week is just as beneficial. Just keep the journal by your bedside or carry it with you so that you can keep track of things that you may forget. Express thanks for the unexpected blessings that come your way.
- Upon rising in the morning, take a few moments to notice all the good in your life and be grateful for these blessings. Whisper or shout an enthusiastic, "I am grateful for this day!"
- Laugh often. Opt for romantic comedies over violent or horror films. Let your silliness show.
- Spend time in community, and allow your soul to shine with the help of others.

THINK

Summary

Become an agent of change.

- Challenge yourself to move out of your comfort zone and effect change.
- Come from love in all your actions and positive change will follow.
- Figure out your *why* and become intrinsically motivated.
- Fill your life with optimists and people who inspire you.
- Affirm your mission and vision daily.

Grow your confidence to effect long-lasting change.

- Know that you are enough: you are worthy, you are whole.
- Talk to yourself as you would talk to someone you love.
- Be aware of when you are in a negative mindset, and get your *but* out of the way.
- Be consistent in all you do; show up for life and show your integrity.
- When performing any task, be aware and fully present.

How we eat and move affects our brains, which impacts how we feel every day.

- Neurotransmitters are chemicals in your brain that, when balanced, help you feel happy, healthy, at peace, and focused.
- When hormones and neurotransmitters work together in balance, your body functions at top performance.
- Mirror neurons mimic what is around us, so peopling our lives with positive influences is important. And expressing our best influences positivity in those around us.
- Be it to see it and see it to be it.
- Practice meditation to increase concentration, peace of mind, and healthy immunity, and to decrease stress and loneliness.

Happiness is an important part of health and thriving in life.

- Irrevocable happiness does not depend on any outside conditions or circumstances. Discover what brings you ultimate joy.
- Happiness is a core value; you can be a happy person even when life brings grief or sadness.
- Laugh as often as possible.
- Be in community and shift your focus from "me" to "we."
- Practice gratitude daily to elevate your thinking and motivate positive change.

Part II

· · · · · · · · · ·

EAT

PART II

Now I see the secret of making the best person:
it is to grow in the open air
and to eat and sleep with the earth.

—Walt Whitman

Typical diets typically fail, and most diets are not sustainable as a life-style. Americans especially have a love-hate relationship with diets, and for many, it can be a self-sabotaging addiction: we hate to go on them, and we love to get off them. Unsatisfied, we then try the next latest fad, and the vicious cycle goes on and on while our confidence wanes. Let's face it: if diets worked, Americans would be the fittest and healthiest people on the planet, but clearly we are not.

At any given time, you can find around sixty thousand books related to dieting. Whether you want to lose ten pounds in a weekend, mainline animal-based proteins until the cows come home, or never have to touch another vegetable, chances are someone has written a how-to diet book on whatever diet you choose. You can have meals delivered right to your home, measured and complete, with shelf lives longer than your own life expectancy. There are thousands of solutions being promised, yet we are fatter than ever; more depressed than ever; and seeking more surgeries, magic potions, and pills to "fix" us than ever.

Think Eat Move Thrive (TEMT) is not a restrictive diet, nor does it hand you a magic pill. You will not be on this diet to reach a desired out-come only to get off it as soon as you can. Yo-yo dieting is one of the worst things you can do to your body and your health. Why? Because yo-yo diet-ing and weight cycling have a negative impact on your heart, metabolism, blood sugar, blood pressure, and immunity. It may also lead to increased inflammation in the body, increased risk of death from cardiovascular disease, and poor circulation.[1] The TEMT Program, on the other hand, is our habitual, everyday way of eating and living; there is no end point. It's a complete life-wellness program that becomes your new norm—a way to Thrive everyday. The TEMT Program is not about a specific diet in the usual sense of the word; it's about a living diet from the perspective and true origin of the Latin word *diaeta*, which means "way of life."

We are going to dig in to food together. We want you to know how, why, what, and when you should be eating to give you joy, fulfillment, and vitality. We have had the honor and enlightening experience of learning, coaching, and witnessing what makes for a near-ideal eating lifestyle. The TEMT Program is the result of all that we've learned about healthy, balanced eating—a program that we've taken several thousand patients through to reclaim their health and their true selves.

The TEMT Program is a perspective on eating that enables you to tap back into your body's innate wisdom and enables you to experience physiological, psychological, and emotional levels of unlimited flourishing. By leveraging the power of habit and intrinsic motivation, you can sustain the desire to nurture your body with healing foods.

When you become conscious of the way you feel—emotionally and physically—before and after you eat or drink certain foods, you will begin to eat with the end experience in mind. You will choose nutrient-dense, whole foods rather than overprocessed, nutrient-void, calorie-dense foods because you will notice a difference in how you feel and function as a result of your choices.

Eating with the end in mind supports us in making choices about food that build a more confident, optimistic, centered, and energized body and brain chemistry. This type of chemistry encourages us to wake up every day and be ready to express our innate awesomeness. With TEMT, you will be on your way to feeling, being, and expressing greatness like never before.

Are you ready to eat? Are you willing to feel and look your best? Time to step in and step up. It's time to eat!

Dr. James on EAT:
http://youtu.be/DLTJ2GcmFec

5

Why EAT

Many of us have lost sight of why we eat. Of course, the obvious answer is that we eat to sustain life. Sometimes we eat because we're bored, lonely, sad, angry; or sheer habit tells us to put something in our mouth. But eating and preparing food should be enjoyed and celebrated. It should help us Thrive, not just survive. It is a daily ritual that can be spiritual and holy as well as satisfying, creative, and fun; yet we often eat with little or no thought about what and how much we put in our mouths. It's time to remember how to eat with intention—to discover why we eat and what it means to Thrive.

Your Life as the First Course

While we can assure you that we will get to the "meat and bones" of the TEMT Program and food, we want to take a little bit of time now to talk about what truly feeds us. Yes, of course, food feeds us literally. But look around your life. What else feeds you? Family, friends, career, sports, hobbies, all of the above?

We are inspired by the integrative nutrition work and philosophy of Joshua Rosenthal—in particular, his work on primary and secondary foods. In his book *Integrative Nutrition*, he states, "Primary food is more than what is on your plate. Healthy relationships, regular physical activity, a fulfilling career, and a rich and dedicated spiritual practice can fill your soul and satisfy your hunger for life. When primary food is balanced and satiating, your life feeds you, making what you eat secondary."[1] Read that one more time. Let the statement and its powerful truth wash over you.

Think about a time when you were out of touch with eating. Maybe you've always been. When we are stressed or feeling disconnected from family or friends, or when we are not aligned with our personal integrity and purpose, we are very vulnerable to making poor food choices. How do you tend to eat when you are feeling lonely or less than your best? Do you desire comfort from food? Do you notice that no matter what or how much you eat, you almost never feel satisfied?

Take this one step further and think about when you are connecting with the primary foods that nourish your soul and life. Do you feel purposeful and fully connected? Are you serving and loving yourself and those around you with your best? Being in integrity with your life's choices feeds you. You gain energy and confidence when you are plugged in to what truly and deeply nourishes you.

When your primary foods are feeding your soul, what do you feed your body—nourishing, nutrient-dense whole foods? If your primary foods leave you unfulfilled, sad, stressed, empty, or angry, what happens with the secondary foods? Do sugar, carbohydrates, unhealthy fats, and salt draw you in? We have witnessed what happens when you live in alignment with what truly feeds you first, and we can tell you: this primary food practice serves as a foundation for making impeccable choices with the secondary foods.

To lay the foundation for TEMT eating, look at your life as it stands today. Does your present occupation support you, not just financially but emotionally? Whatever you need to do to make your relationship with your job feel good, become meaningful, and fulfill you, make those changes now. If there is no flexibility, it is time to reevaluate your current role. How about your relationships? Remember the idea of peopling your life well, and put that in action.

Every morning before breakfast, set an intention to be present to your highest potential—your vision for your best living. Nourish this healthy beginning with foods that will feed this intention. Throughout the day, acknowledge if you are craving junk and notice when you may be off your game. Look within to see where you can realign and refocus your light and love with positive rituals and courageous action, rather than empty calories.

• • • • • • • • • • • •

ACTION STEP
Think about the following questions:
What triggers your cravings?
How can you proactively participate in nourishing healthy beginnings?
What are three rituals that you can engage in immediately or create to support healthy beginnings each day?
Consider these suggestions:

- Create a signature breakfast smoothie that you know you can enjoy when either lack of creativity or lack of time interferes with your breakfast plans.
- Keep track of what you eat in the morning and how you feel throughout the afternoon. You'll learn whether or not what you are eating in the morning supports your greatness or not.
- Jump-start your day with warm water and lemon (and a dash of cayenne pepper). This is a great ritual that stimulates and strengthens the immune system, digestive system, and kidneys, and does wonders for the skin.

- Begin the day with meditation. Although this isn't an eating ritual, meditation will actually create a chemistry and a mindset to set you up for healthy beginnings that last all day long.

• • • • • • • • • • • •

 Primary Versus Secondary Nutrition
http://www.youtube.com/watch?v=iboG-pE9zi_Y&list=PLDF26DC5254801299

Your Eating Personality

Do your eating habits reflect your essential self? What is your present relationship with food? Do you use it to support your personal mission and vision? Is food something that you think about only when you're hungry, serving more of a utilitarian purpose? Do you ever find yourself using food to satisfy and fill a void? If so, does food ever truly fill it? These are all interesting questions, but what does your eating personality actually say about you?

We know that eating is a physiological need, but there is a large psychological and emotional component to eating. Let's look back for a moment at our section on "I Am Enough" in Part I. When we come from an emotional place of chronic not enoughness, we tend to overeat to fill the void. Do you eat because you're hungry for approval, recognition, or companionship? Recognizing our psychological triggers is the first step in determining our eating personality.

We've listed and described eight dominant eating personalities below. Read each one and see which one resonates with you. Maybe you don't want or need to alter your eating personality, but if you do, we've given you ideas and strategies for achieving balance in spite of or in celebration of your eating personality.

1. **Emotional Eater:** You use food for comfort, turning to food when you're sad, lonely, needy, stressed out, procrastinating, or avoiding something. It is not unusual to occasionally turn to food for comfort, but when it becomes a daily habit, it's time to address the deeper issues. The causes of emotional eating can be pretty deep—more than we can cover here. We are big proponents of journaling to keep track of not just the food you are eating but the triggers as well. Another option is counseling, to establish new tools—other than food—for coping. Daily exercise, even just fifteen to twenty minutes daily, can also help to balance the emotions that are driving unconscious eating.

2. **Trendy Eater:** You follow all the latest food fads—Paleo one month, raw food the next; then the juice cleanse, Zone, macrobiotic, vegan, Atkins, South Beach—but you haven't really found one that you've stayed with for the long haul. We can certainly relate to this eating personality; we've admittedly experimented with every diet we just listed. It can be fun to try out and be a part of the latest craze, but when we get too obsessed with eating in such a restrictive way, we lose some of the joy and natural instinct that goes along with simply eating well. Also, many of you may be using these diets for fast weight loss or for the general purpose of only losing weight. When we eat for health, we're much more likely to stick with the program. To balance out the fascination (and perhaps obsession) with the latest and greatest health trends, focus on an overall healthy relationship with food. Use the TEMT Program to get an expansive and comprehensive idea of how to enjoy a diverse range of healthy foods.

3. **Scarcity Eater:** You may have experienced a shortage of food when you were growing up, or food may have been used as a punishment or reward. You may have experienced longer periods of hunger than

others in your peer group. This personality eats almost everything in sight out of fear that there won't be enough. Try to recognize where the behavior is coming from and assess your current situation. If food scarcity is a real issue for you, then support is available across the country through food banks, churches, schools, and other charitable organizations. If you have plenty of food but you struggle with managing the amount that you eat, practice moderation in situations where food is freely available, including buffets, office parties, and dinner parties. The best strategy we've come across is to first choose a smaller plate. Then stop eating before you feel full, to prevent overeating (practice mindfulness, and learn to become aware of your stomach feeling full and satisfied). Learning to become aware of your physical satisfaction—and why or what you're truly eating for—creates a base for "I have enough" contentment.

4. **Mindless Eater:** You don't really think about the foods that cross your lips. Fast food is a regular part of your life; and you eat in your car, in front of the television, or at your desk, as there's a perceived belief of convenience and time limits. You haven't made healthy food a part of your life—the hallmark of someone who is overscheduled or not taking enough time. To balance this personality, schedule time for relaxation and reflection. Make time to prepare healthy meals and snacks before you head out for the day so that you will not be tempted to "drive thru" anywhere on your way home. Make health a priority, and take charge of your time and commitment. Take steps to simply focus on eating: enjoy your interaction with food. Step away from the computer or the television when it's time to eat your lunch or dinner.

5. **Mindful Nature Worshipper:** Eating is as much a sociopolitical and environmental statement as it is an effort to always do the right thing. You only eat organic produce and very limited animal prod-

ucts, but when you do, they are always certified humanely raised, free range, and grass fed. And you take time to enjoy your food, away from distractions. If this describes your eating personality, good for you. The plus side of this eating personality is that it is more nutrient dense, nourishing, and usually results in fewer diet-related health issues. The best way to balance this way of eating is to check in with yourself to make sure that your eating stays intuitive and doesn't get stressful. Sometimes, trying to be too perfect with your diet can actually add stress, which will undo some of the positive benefits of mindful eating.

6. **Junk-Food Junkie:** You keep junk food stashed all over the place—at home, in your car, in your desk drawer at work. You'll eat whatever is handy and quick, and it's usually salty or sweet. Sometimes this personality can mimic the Emotional Eater, who reaches for comfort food on a whim. Balance it by adding more structure, fruits, and vegetables to your life. Plan ahead by eating a healthy breakfast, packing a nourishing lunch, and stepping away from whatever you are doing when a craving arises. A quick walk around the block or the office, or a five-minute timeout can do wonders for cravings.

7. **Starve All Day, Night Binger:** You're pressed for time in the morning or you're just not a breakfast person. You drink a few cups of coffee or tea, and you're too busy for lunch. You get home famished after work, and you don't stop eating from the time you walk in the door to the time your head hits the pillow. Unfortunately, this is one of the worst habits that we can develop. It sets the stage for erratic blood sugar levels and wreaks havoc on your metabolism. The body stores fat all day because it thinks it's in starvation mode, and you're setting yourself up for less-than-brilliant choices once you walk through the door. Unless you have a loving partner waiting to welcome you home with a healthy dinner, chances are you're going to

go for the bag of chips, box of crackers, log of cheese, bottle of wine, or all of the above. Balance this personality by making yourself and breakfast a priority. Breakfast is non-negotiable in the TEMT Program, as it is an essential component for thriving all day, every day. Another tip is to stay hydrated with fresh water throughout the day.

8. **Habitual Eater (aka Finicky):** You eat the same thing every day. For breakfast, it's oatmeal. For lunch, it's a salad with grilled chicken. And for dinner, it's a piece of fish with rice and vegetables. You snack on raw almonds and have a banana every day. Okay, admittedly this may sound like the healthy version of being a habitual eater, but remember this is just an example. Variety is key for a well-rounded, healthy lifestyle. If stepping outside your food comfort zone causes anxiety, there may be cause for seeking further support via counseling or therapy. Rotating foods, fruits, vegetables, proteins, and grains is essential for getting the variety of nutrition that we need. Consider adding just one new food every day or every other day, be it a fruit or a vegetable, a new nut or seed, or a different protein source.

Author Check-In

Debra's eating personality: James and I both straddle between being Trendy Eaters and Habitual Eaters. As we've mentioned before, there aren't many diets we haven't experimented with—the exception being Atkins, since neither of us are big meat eaters. James simply knows what foods work well for his body and brain, and he rarely veers from those foods. His habitual eating has occasionally become a problem when he's overdone too much of good thing. That's when I remind him to rotate more foods into the mix. Salmon, kale, and eggs are all examples of foods he has had to take out of his diet at one time or another and gradually rotate back in. He is not one to crave junk food or eat mindlessly. I tend to be a habitual eater as well but have definitely juggled the habits of an Emotional Eater and a Trendy Eater. When I was younger and had less of a handle on how food and exercise choices impacted my hormones and emotions, I had more of an emotionally driven eating personality. I still notice how emotions can drive my cravings: when I'm sad, I don't eat as much; when happy or hyper, I may eat more than normal; when grounded and centered, I make very balanced choices.

Remember that these eight eating personalities are only examples. You might be an exact description of one of them or a combination of two or three. And these eating personalities are not absolute or stagnant; you may move from one to another depending on your life situation or emotional state of mind. The key to this practice of identifying your eating personality is to bring to light the what, why, and how of your eating habits. Being clearly informed is a must if you want to become an intentional and mindful eater, and it empowers you to make new choices that better serve your goals. Putting food to work for you is an enlightening ritual, and choosing foods that support your highest expression can be fortifying and fulfilling. Fortunately, we will be taking the guesswork out of this for you when it comes to food and TEMT.

Exercise: Feed Your Soul

Think about what feeds your soul (aside from food). It may be friendships, art, sports, family, career, or a combination of one or more interests. Is it possible that your eating personality intersects with the things that nurture your soul? Think about it. If you are a Junk-Food Junkie and art feeds your soul, do you associate the two? If you are an artist, do you often have a sugar stash nearby? If you are a lover of art, do you feel better observing art when you are eating candy or popcorn, or drinking alcohol? If so, it is time to make some new associations. This exercise is about linking your primary "food"—what feeds your soul—with healthy habits.

Part II: EAT

Take out a journal and write down your primary foods. Next to that, write down how those primary foods contribute to your eating personality. You may or may not find an association. If you do, it may be a really positive association. For example, you may have written that your primary food is friendships, and your friends are health nuts who encourage you to eat wonderful, healthy foods. This is a positive association compared to a primary food that is one's career—a career that causes you to starve yourself all day and stuff yourself at night. This is more of a negative association because when you fail to nourish your body all day, your performance and productivity suffer; your confidence and mood are nowhere near where they could be if you made yourself a priority by simply eating a healthy breakfast and lunch.

6

EAT Outcomes

Our lifestyles and eating choices impact nearly every aspect of our lives, but in particular, these choices directly impact our health and well-being. Poor choices lead to increased inflammation in the body, and the SAD (Standard American Diet) drives inflammation. Refined carbohydrates, sugar, trans fats, empty calories, fiberless foods, and an imbalance of unhealthy fats (partially hydrogenated oils, trans fats, and fried foods) encourage inflammation. Being overweight and sedentary increases inflammation. But what does inflammation actually mean, and why do our TEMT diet choices focus on dousing the flames?

Chronic inflammation is almost always brought on by poor lifestyle choices or choices that simply do not work with your unique biochemistry. Symptoms include fatigue, insomnia, aches, pains, skin issues, weight gain, irritability, weakened or over-reactive immune response, digestive issues; or simply feeling bad, chronically older than you are, weaker than you should be, and looking like you are aging faster. Over time, inflammation left unchecked will lead to a much more destructive and potentially fatal situation. By altering and improving food choices, we can reverse inflammation and the damage it causes.

The Inflammation Epidemic

We are in the midst of an inflammation epidemic in the United States. A consistent state of inflammation can be likened to smoldering embers on a fire: feed it a little, and the flame will rage; douse it a bit, and it goes back to smoldering. Increased consumption of processed foods; genetically modified organisms (GMOs), toxins, and chemicals in our food supply; and sedentary lifestyles have combined to create this current catastrophe of chronic disease, all relative to inflammation.

From heart disease to type 2 diabetes, depression to Alzheimer's, the relationship between chronic inflammation, disease, and premature death is sobering. The SAD diet—high in sugar, refined starches, and trans fats and low in fiber and omega-3 fatty acids—contributes to the production of inflammatory chemicals that increase the risk of these chronic diseases.[1] SAD fuels inflammation; TEMT cools it down. The main dietary strategy of TEMT includes a generous consumption of vegetables; moderate consumption of fruits, nuts, seeds, whole grains, lean proteins, and omega-3 fatty acids; and little consumption of saturated fat. Our strategy is in line with the Mediterranean, Okinawan, and anti-inflammatory dietary principles, which are consistent with decreased inflammation.

The inflammation that is silently debilitating millions of lives every day is subtle and insidious. The latest statistics from the Centers for Disease Control (CDC) list the prevalence of obesity (in 2011–2012) at over one-third of adults in the United States (roughly 35 percent). During this time period, over 78 million American adults and 12.5 million adolescents and children were obese.[2] Nearly 2 million Americans were diagnosed with diabetes in 2010;[3] chronic arthritis affects an estimated 50 million American adults;[4] and over 5 million Americans have

Alzheimer's disease.[5] What all of these diseases have in common is that they originate from chronic, systemic inflammation. Chronic inflammation breaks down the body and immune system over time, and incites disease. It contributes to the failure of mind and body and fast-forwards the aging process, leaving you weak, depressed, and more susceptible to a host of life-threatening diseases.

The typical SAD delivers too many calories and not enough nutrition, thus encouraging inflammation. When our eating is out of balance—when we're eating a lot of fast, processed, and fried foods; excess sugar; and drinking excess alcohol—a cascade of inflammatory prostaglandins (hormone-like compounds) are created, triggering inflammation in the body.

Our bodies are designed to support homeostasis, which is a state of dynamic balance. This includes being able to sustain a healthy balance of pro- and anti-inflammatory states of being. We have thrived for thousands of years with this innate and beautiful chemistry, as our diets have been, for the most part, balanced in nature and practice. In the last century, and really the last few decades, our diets have become based on more convenience and fast food, and we have tipped the balance toward pro-inflammatory compounds.

With this new and unfortunate reality, it would appear we are doomed as chronic disease rates increase like never before; rare diseases experience a resurgence; feelings of depression, fatigue, and hopelessness abound; and we die way before our time from preventable diseases.

Top Ten Foods to Avoid

1. Potato chips
2. Donuts
3. Packaged baked goods
4. Margarine

5. High-fructose corn syrup and artificial sweeteners like sucralose and aspartame
6. Energy drinks
7. Hot dogs and lunch meat that contain nitrites/nitrates
8. Movie theatre popcorn (trans fats, excess sodium, artificial coloring, flavoring, GMOs [genetically modified organisms])
9. Nonorganic corn and soy products—almost always GMO
10. Artificial colors and flavors

• • • • • • • • • • • • •

ACTION STEP

Examine your pantry and refrigerator, and see where there is room for improvement. Remove any foods that do not truly nourish and sustain your total well-being. Get rid of cookies; donuts; crackers; and all things containing high-fructose corn syrup (HFCS), artificial sweeteners, coloring, trans fats (anything containing partially hydrogenated oils), and other ingredients that you can't pronounce. Stop making excuses for why you can't throw them away or why you brought them into your home in the first place.

After you've completed the purge, it's time to restock with foods that support the anti-inflammatory pathways in the body. Add dark-green leafy vegetables like broccoli, chard, and kale; yellow veggies like squash and cauliflower (yes, we know it's white); raw nuts like walnuts, almonds, macadamia nuts, and pecans; and seeds like pumpkin, chia, hemp, and flax. Add whole grains like quinoa, amaranth, oats, brown rice, and wild rice. Add high-antioxidant spices like turmeric, curry, ginger, rosemary, oregano, thyme, and cinnamon; and enjoy pure dark cocoa in moderation to soothe your body and soul. All of these strategies will help put out the fire.

· · · · · · · · · · · ·

Nutrient-Dense Eating

The TEMT Program is plant based and nutrient dense. Nutrient-dense foods pack the greatest amount of nutrition in the smallest packages. In other words, these are foods that contain high amounts of vitamins, minerals, antioxidants, phytonutrients, and essential fatty acids while containing relatively few calories. Fruits and vegetables are the most obvious examples. Dark-green leafy vegetables, cruciferous vegetables (cauliflower, cabbage, kale, Brussels sprouts, mustard greens, broccoli), berries, and cherries are all nutrient-dense power foods. Nutrient-dense foods deliver high nutrition and low drama.

But we cannot live on nutrient-dense foods alone. If we did, our diets would be too low in healthy fats and likely too low in calories as well. In addition to nutrient-dense foods like fruits, vegetables, and whole grains, we encourage nuts and seeds, cold-water fish, legumes, beans, and small amounts of sustainably raised animal products. For vegetarians or vegans, we would suggest adding small amounts of organic, fermented soy. And while we know for certain that some authorities will beg to differ when it comes to adding grains to the diet, we know that in the happiest communities where people live the longest, this is how people eat.

 Antioxidants and Optimism
http://www.youtube.com/watch?v=1FkY8O7HUxg&list=PLDF2 6DC5254801299

What About Wine?

You may be wondering if alcohol—specifically wine—fits into a healthy, vital, and anti-inflammatory lifestyle. It does in moderation. Red wine is a great source of resveratrol, a powerful polyphenol antioxidant. Resveratrol may offer supportive benefits in insulin sensitivity, which is important for metabolism, heart health, and the prevention of type 2 diabetes. And it has been referred to as a miracle antiaging remedy.[6] Several studies have revealed that resveratrol has a broad range of other health benefits, including protection against atherosclerosis, many forms of cancer, as well as neurodegenerative diseases.[7]

One challenge with resveratrol is in the absorption of it into your bloodstream. A simple, fun, and truly delicious way to augment resveratrol's bang for its buck is to take a sip of red wine (or grape juice) and then swish it around in your mouth for a full minute before you swallow it. This will help assimilate its benefits into your bloodstream, where it can do its good.

We find the largest population of healthy, long-lived adults in Okinawa, Japan. The traditional Okinawan diet consists of sweet potatoes, green and yellow vegetables, legumes, and a small amount of fish and pork. Okinawans receive plenty of natural exercise and sunlight through gardening, and they stop eating when they are about 80 percent full. They also eat little to no dairy products or eggs.

The Mediterranean diet differs slightly from the Okinawan in a few key areas. Dairy products (mostly yogurt and cheese), unrefined grains, wine (usually red), and olive oil play a major to moderate role. Like the Okinawan diet, the Mediterranean diet (patterned after those living in Greece and Southern Italy) includes a high consumption of fruits and vegetables, a moderate consumption of fish, and a low consumption of meat. Mediterranean residents are probably most widely known for their use and consumption of olive oil, which is naturally high in antioxidants and has anti-inflammatory properties. We use olive oil almost exclusively now (in addition to coconut oil), and we'll talk a bit more about the Mediterranean diet shortly.

Anti-inflammatory diets have been written about and numerous experts have touted the benefits, each giving their own spin on what an anti-inflammatory diet looks like. We're guilty of this too, teaching our own version of an anti-inflammatory lifestyle for nearly twenty years. What we can all probably agree on is that plant foods and the phytochemicals that they contain decrease inflammation in the body. As we've shared, inflammation is one of the primary causes (if not *the* primary cause) of most modern-day chronic diseases.

An anti-inflammatory diet is quite similar to the Okinawan and Mediterranean diets; it just hasn't been defined so specifically. In other words, there is no exact definition, but there are several interpretations. The foods we recommend in TEMT and the foods that make up the bulk of our 30-day program are in line with the best practices of Okinawan, Mediterranean, and anti-inflammatory philosophies, combined with our years of personal and professional research and experience. This includes plenty of vegetables and fruits (we recommend at least seven [ideally nine] servings daily [mostly vegetable]); omega-3 fats from cold-water fish; walnuts, chia, hemp, and flax seeds; sesame seeds, Brussels sprouts, and cauliflower. We recommend the elimination of refined grains like white rice, white potatoes, white flour, and all white-flour products and pastas (made from white or seminola flour). Whole grains like brown rice, quinoa, barley, amaranth, oats, and sprouted grains are all part of our anti-inflammatory plan. And spices like ginger, turmeric, curry, cinnamon, cayenne, and garlic are all part of the TEMT Program. Of course, adding olive oil, avocado, and coconut oil (to a lesser degree) and eliminating all partially hydrogenated (trans fatty acids) fats is equally essential to the anti-inflammatory lifestyle and TEMT. While this doesn't include every ingredient in our program, it should give you an idea of what forms the basis of TEMT.

Eat Your Greens

What the TEMT Program and the Okinawan, Mediterranean, and anti-inflammatory diets have in common is plenty of dietary fiber, monounsaturated fat, lean and clean protein, and powerful phytonutrients that are naturally abundant in plant-based diets.

When you settle for the SAD way of eating, you tend to be overfed yet undernourished. To thrive and achieve optimum wellness, vegetables are non-negotiable—so we want you to connect to a more plant-based diet. The greater the quantity and variety of vegetables and fruits in your diet, the lower the incidence and risk for having a heart attack, experiencing a stroke, and contracting cancer.

Vegan Protein Alternatives to Soy

In recent years, the true benefits of a soy-rich diet have come into question, leaving many vegans and vegetarians wondering where to turn next for protein. Contrary to what you might hear, there are a number of vegetarian, soy-alternative protein sources: adzuki beans, almonds, black beans, fava beans, kidney beans, lentils, garbanzo beans, mung beans, peanuts, pecans, pinto beans, split peas, walnuts, white beans, yard-long beans.

What do we have against soy? Having been vegans for many years, we've certainly eaten our fair share of soy. When we were in school it was still thought of as one of the most versatile and healthy foods available. Twenty years later, we now know that there are downsides to eating soy, in particular, unfermented soy. Soy has become ubiquitous in the American food supply. It's in everything from infant formulas to meat patties and vegetarian "meat substitute" food items. Consumption of unfermented soy has been linked to infertility (male and female),[8] thyroid issues,[9] digestive problems, and even Alzheimer's disease.[10] Currently over 90 percent of the US soy fields are planted with genetically modified (GM) soy (and a large percentage of that is going into animal feed). If you are not eating organic soy (or organic dairy and animal products), chances are very likely that you are getting genetically modified soy on a regular basis. Soaking, fermentation, and heating soy foods may decrease the adverse effects of consuming soy.[11]

Note: We do not include wheat gluten (seitan) as an option here because, quite frankly, we don't like it; it's like poison for anyone sensitive to gluten. However, if you know you don't have an issue with gluten, seitan may be a viable protein alternative for you. We just haven't personally or professionally experienced individuals thriving on it.

To clarify, we are not saying that everyone should become vegan; we are strongly suggesting plant-based or plant-focused eating. And don't worry; you will not become protein deficient. A protein-deficient American is virtually unheard of, even though this is a common misconception about eating plant based. As a frame of reference (and to support your plant-based peace of mind), let's look at comparing the protein amounts in broccoli versus steak. There are approximately 5.4 grams of protein in 100 calories of steak. There are approximately 11.2 grams of protein in 100 calories of broccoli. Per calorie, broccoli delivers nearly twice as much on the protein front, and a plant-based protein is more anti-inflammatory compared to animal-based proteins.

If just the thought of letting go of red meat makes you feel like a plant-based lifestyle isn't for you, we'd like you to consider something:

if meat eaters ate less than half a serving of red meat each day, deaths would drop by roughly 8 percent.[12] If you choose to eat meat, you have the choice of consuming healthier meat. Look for meat from grass-fed cattle or buffalo, grain-fed poultry, and animals who are humanely raised (free range) and slaughtered. These meats are healthier, containing less saturated fat and more health-promoting fatty acids, such as conjugated linoleic acid (CLA). CLA may help to reduce body fat and improve immune function. So, just think about what you're eating when you do choose to eat meat, and make sure you are having plenty of veggies on the side. You will Thrive.

Meat and Mortality

A study supported by the National Institutes of Health concluded that people who consumed the highest levels of both unprocessed and processed red meat had the highest risk of dying from all-causes, including cancer and heart disease. One additional daily serving of unprocessed red meat increased risk of death by 13 percent, and an additional daily serving of processed red meat (lunch meat, sausage, bacon, hot dogs, etc.) increased the risk by 20 percent.[13]

Phytochemicals (*phyto* means "plant") are naturally occurring anti-oxidants in plants. A plant-focused diet helps us to Thrive by

1. serving as our first line of defense against disease, aging, and inflammation;
2. keeping healthy watch over the genes that promote inflammation;
3. reducing the risk of stroke;
4. supporting heart health and helping to fight heart disease on multiple fronts (for example, eating plant foods reduces platelet aggregation

and the stickiness of your platelets; the less sticky your platelets the better and healthier your circulation);

5. supporting healthy cholesterol and blood lipid levels;
6. improving cholesterol profile; and
7. helping to reduce blood pressure.

 Dr. James on Plant-Based Protein
http://youtu.be/jLfeFSK8lwc

Sugar and Aging

It probably isn't new information that our consumption of sugar has increased considerably in the last few hundred years. There are many conflicting statistics out there, but basically, at the turn of the twentieth century, Americans were consuming under 10 pounds of sugar per person on an annual basis. By 1913, that increased dramatically to about 76 pounds per person. Today, the average American consumes about 150 to 170 pounds of sugar in a year.[14]

Liquid Sugar

Soda is the leading source of added dietary sugars. Other sweetened beverages, like sports drinks and specialty coffee drinks, are also contributing a substantial amount of sugar to our current addiction. The average amount of sugar in one soda is 33 grams to 35 grams. The average energy drink has about 50 grams of sugar. The added calories from drinking one soda (or one specialty coffee drink) every day can add 15 pounds to your frame by the end of the year.

Sugar isn't sweet when it comes to our skin or looking, feeling, and being vibrant. You can Botox your way out of a few wrinkles, but if you continue to over-sugar your life, wrinkles will eventually win out. Enjoying too much sugar encourages something called advanced glycation end products (AGEs), and these sweet villains are all about driving disease and premature aging. AGEs are formed when sugar mixes with amino acids. This creates the perfect environment for inflammation, disease, aging, and premature death. The formation of AGEs has been linked to an increased risk for (you've guessed it) heart disease, type 2 diabetes, and Alzheimer's disease. When you limit and avoid sugar, you starve the AGEs formation process. And guess what else happens? Beauty increases, energy increases, life expectancy increases, and thriving happens!

Of all the molecules that can inflict damage on your mind and body, sugar is one of the worst. Sugar encourages fat deposits around your vital organs (this is a keynote of heart disease and type 2 diabetes); and it drives inflammation, which increases insulin and leptin levels while decreasing the sensitivity to both of these vital hormones. As this insensitivity becomes chronic, we fast-forward the aging process and increase the risks for metabolic syndrome, obesity, type 2 diabetes, heart disease, and cancer.

It is normal for blood sugar levels to rise a bit after a meal; however, it is not normal—or healthy—to have blood sugar levels remain elevated for a long period of time afterward. Too many Americans have created a situation where their blood sugar is chronically and permanently elevated. This chronic elevation makes us overweight, tired, depressed, and sick. Are you ready to feel better and kick the sugar addiction?

Kicking the sugar habit is a life-giving, life-changing decision. What is your *why* for letting go of sugar? Notice when you tend to crave sugar. Is it when you are you watching TV, hanging out with certain people, doing things that you do not enjoy? Be mindful of how sugar finds its sneaky way into your daily routine, and watch for the subtle triggers that initiate its desire.

How to Maintain a Balanced Sugar Level

- Do not skip meals.
- Eat a small meal or snack at least every three hours to maintain balanced blood sugar levels.
- Healthfully and proactively manage stress, as stress drives sugar cravings. Chronic stress decreases serotonin and, in turn, encourages the desire for sugar, and processed and refined carbs.
- Always have a protein-rich breakfast, and eat within thirty minutes to an hour of waking up. This will help prevent binging later in the day.
- Exercise religiously. Strength training increases insulin sensitivity (drives sugar from the blood into the muscle), which decreases sugar cravings and encourages fat metabolism, lean muscle building, overall sustained energy, mental clarity, and high-level well-being.

Your best bet when it comes to cutting down on sugar in the diet is to stick to fresh vegetables and fruits, and steer clear of added sugars—especially packaged foods and processed sugars (including corn syrup and high-fructose corn syrup). Sugar has insidiously found its way into every packaged good on the shelf. One teaspoon of sugar, or 4 grams, equals approximately 16 calories. To figure out how much sugar is in one serving of whatever you are eating or drinking, just do the math: if the product lists 20 grams of sugar, then that means it contains 5 teaspoons of sugar, or 80 sugar-derived calories. Aim to keep total sugar for the day at or below 10 percent of your total caloric intake. So if you are consuming 1,800 calories daily, no more than 180 calories (45 grams) are sugars.

The Multiple Identities of Sugar

Sugar comes in many disguises and goes by many different names. There are literally dozens (if not hundreds) of names for sugar that you will commonly find on ingredient labels. Here is a short sample: brown rice syrup, maple syrup, honey, agave nectar, dextrose, sucrose, glucose, corn syrup, high-fructose corn syrup, fructose, cane sugar, barley malt, galactose, maltose, molasses, maltodextrin, dehydrated cane juice. Start reading labels and look for foods that you eat regularly that may contain hidden sources of added sugar.

It is challenging to keep your daily sugar at or under 10 percent, so you may want to write things down at first to keep track. Again, remember the math: for every 1,000 calories you consume, no more than 100 calories (25 grams) should come from added sugars. That's less than the amount of sugar found in a tall Starbucks Caramel Frappuccino, which contains 45 grams of sugar! Many sweetened yogurts, cereals, juices, smoothies, and snack bars contain a lot of sugar, so if you aren't already reading nutritional facts on product labels, it's time to start!

 Sugar and Your Skin
http://www.youtube.com/watch?v=HnBh5WarrI4&list=PLDF2 6DC5254801299

Do I Need to Detox?

We are often asked for our opinions on cleansing and detox programs. Though it's not a cut-and-dry answer, we do believe that periodic cleansing is a smart idea if you want to really Thrive. We usually recommend cleansing with the change of seasons or at least a few times a year. When we refer to cleansing, what we really mean is super clean eating. True fasting, like only consuming water for a length of time, is something that should be done under the supervision of a qualified health professional (with the blessing of your primary care doctor). There is a time and a place for fasting or modified fasting, but that isn't the purpose of TEMT. The good news is that the TEMT Program is a very clean-eating program to begin with; if you commit to the TEMT style of eating, you'll be in great shape. However, even a tobacco- and alcohol-free, 100 percent organic lifestyle cannot protect us from environmental exposure to toxins.

In the United States and across the planet, we are overcome and enveloped by toxins, literally marinating in a toxic stew that is playing a major role in our present disease crisis. But you only eat vegan, organic foods? We wish we could tell you that you're safe from toxins, but the truth is, exposure to environmental toxins—from nonstick skillets and electromagnetic frequencies (EMFs) to can linings, and from the air we breathe to the water we drink—is nearly unavoidable. And that's why it may help to give your body a break every once in a while, to at least decrease the toxic burden and recharge all your vital organs.

Author Check-In

James's detox story: About sixteen years ago, I was experiencing severe neurological symptoms. Along with having a few seizures, I began to experience numbness and tingling in my arms and legs; and I suffered from frequent headaches, mild depression, fatigue, and trouble sleeping. All of my symptoms led me to the diagnosis of multiple sclerosis (MS).

Individuals with MS often respond favorably to supplementation with essential fatty acids and fish oils. I am known for my occasional overzealousness; and I'll admit I approached my symptoms with serious zeal in the form of fish for breakfast, fish for lunch, and fish for dinner. I was especially fond of frozen Alaskan halibut and wild salmon burgers, so I would have two of one kind for breakfast and pack two for lunch. Then I'd come home to a fish dinner that Debra lovingly prepared. The more my symptoms flared, the more zealous my fish consumption. It became a vicious circle, because it was likely that some of the fish I was eating contained unsafe levels of mercury.

Finally, I decided I should maybe think about seeing a neurologist—but first, I ran a hair analysis to check for heavy metals. My mercury levels were off the charts! I had never seen results come back so elevated. I formulated a detoxification and chelation (the process of removing heavy metals from the blood-stream) program in partnership with a functional medicine colleague of mine, and let me tell you, detoxing from mercury was neither easy nor fun. But I am happy to say I am now symp-tom free and mercury levels are no longer an issue.

Today, I keep my fish intake in check (no more than once a week), and I will only eat fish that are known to be low mercury carriers. I supplement with fish oils that have been screened and tested for mercury, but I worry about the state of our oceans and how safe our seafood will be, if at all, in the very near future. To keep up on the latest information regarding the safety of seafood consumption, I recommend seafoodwatch .org (from the Monterey Bay Aquarium) and nrdc.org (Natural Resources Defense Council).

So how do we deal with these unavoidable toxins when we are eat-ing as clean and organic as possible? One of the simplest things we can do is to make sure we are drinking plenty of fresh, filtered water. If you don't know the source of your tap water, it is wise to have it tested for possible contaminants like bacteria or heavy metals. It is quite simple (at least it is for a plumber) to install an under-the-sink carbon (or reverse osmosis) water filter that should make your water more than safe and fit to drink, just be sure to change out the filters regularly. We recommend a minimum water consumption of half your weight (in ounces). So for example, if you weigh 150 pounds, you should be drinking at least 75 ounces of water daily, and more if you are working out regularly.

Cleansing and detox programs are all the rage these days; people are juicing, fasting, doing enemas, and having colonics on a regular basis. Some people cleanse to look better (lose weight, improve skin tone, and so on), some want to feel better, and some want both. Many cleansing programs offer a legitimate opportunity for the body to heal and to decrease systemic inflammation; but some cleansing programs may be too extreme and possibly unhealthy—even dangerous. It can become risky when there is a history of drug (prescription or recreational) or alcohol abuse, diabetes, heart disease, or obesity and you decide to cleanse on your own without being monitored by a doctor. We typically don't buy in to the "all or nothing" mentality, meaning, you either starve yourself or you binge eat. Our program is meant to support the body's natural detoxification processes through simple, clean eating. Having said that, we don't mind a few days of juicing to give the body a break from whatever it is you've been feeding it, but we recommend mostly vegetable (as opposed to fruit) juices, diluted 50 percent with pure water, and try to drink something at least every two to three hours to avoid severe drops in blood sugar.

The good news: our bodies are naturally equipped for detoxification; our natural state is not inflamed. Our livers and kidneys are well suited to deal with and discard toxins, and keep us running smooth and clean. When your lifestyle becomes particularly burdensome, or you've lived on the more toxic side of life, it can be helpful and wise to offer your body a bit of extra support in getting itself back into balance and vitality.

Toxicity encourages inflammation. When the toxic burden becomes too great, the liver and kidneys cannot keep up. The result: our liver becomes sluggish and fatty, our kidneys become dysfunctional and inflamed, and we begin the steady decline into toxicity, increasing the likelihood for disease and feeling less than great. When your liver is not functioning at its best, you begin to feel fatigued. An inflamed liver is painfully inefficient at processing sugar, and this doesn't just contribute to weight gain; it also compromises the entire body system. Our cells undergo greater assaults from free radicals, and they are unable to defend themselves.

But toxicity and the subsequent decline in our health, happiness, and well-being doesn't have to be inevitable. You have an opportunity to make simple lifestyle shifts now that will keep your innate, natural detox systems running strong in spite of what is going on around you. The TEMT Program is all about supporting your liver and every organ system in the body.

Never underestimate the power of healthy eating as a way and means to help your body make daily, effective, and healthy detoxification happen. The TEMT eating plan is designed to nourish your natural detoxification systems. More specifically, TEMT naturally raises levels of glutathione, an important antioxidant that plays a major role in detoxification. Glutathione *rules* detoxification.

Glutathione is the queen of the antioxidant army, leading the way in healthy detoxification. We can raise glutathione levels in the body by increasing our intake of cysteine-containing (amino-acid) foods, like broccoli, Brussels sprouts, poultry, yogurt, red peppers, garlic, onions, oats, eggs, and wheat germ. When you are living a more dramatic lifestyle (i.e., excess alcohol, sugar, tobacco, caffeine, processed foods), you deplete glutathione stores. Other foods that build glutathione include whey protein, asparagus, spinach, avocado, squash, melons, grapefruit, and peaches. Antioxidant-rich strawberries, raspberries, kiwi, bell peppers, and mangoes are particularly high in vitamin C, which also feeds glutathione.

If you are the type that likes to jump-start your life with new ways of being, then we recommend a two-week phase-in prior to embarking on the TEMT lifestyle. This looks like eliminating all forms of sugar, artificial sweeteners, alcohol, tobacco, processed foods, fried foods, flour products, and limiting red meat and dairy products. Again, if you have a history of smoking or excessive intake of alcohol, we recommend you work with a doctor who can take you through the process. Of course we are biased towards naturopathic doctors, who are thoroughly trained and skilled in the area of nutrition and dotoxification. To find a registered or licensed naturopathic doctor in your area, visit naturopathic.org and click on "Find a Doctor."

Periodic cleansing is a lifestyle choice that pays dividends beyond looks alone. Like all rituals that support being happy, sexy, and strong, you will be a source of leadership and inspiration for all who witness your commitment to living well. Set the intention and goal to keep your heart focused on the bigger story of your motivation, fueled by your desire to lead and serve. You will have all the fuel you need to keep your inspiration alive and very well!

 Dr. James on Cleansing
http://www.youtube.com/watch?v=vcT-ImNVMYI&list=PLDF26DC5254801299

Exercise: Reclaim Your Kitchen

Three or four times a year, we take time to thoroughly clean house—and this includes food. We're talking about kitchen cabinets, drawers, the refrigerator, and the pantry. Even though we think we're really conscious about the food we bring into the house, it's surprising how much food and snack clutter accumulates. Make it a habit to purge your pantry and refrigerator with the change of seasons. Throw away (or compost) any half-eaten bags of chips or crackers; check the expiration dates on condiments and toss any that have expired; and clean out the vegetable crisper and the cheese drawer (you may be surprised what you find growing at the bottom of the bin!). This is a great opportunity to get rid of the junk food and any other edible distraction that sabotages your mission and vision for your life. Definitely get rid of any products that contain artificial sweeteners, colorings, high-fructose corn syrup, or partially hydrogenated oils.

This exercise is the first step in detoxing your life. Once you've cleared the clutter—the expired, stale, spoiled, and unhealthy foods from your refrigerator and pantry—think about restocking with nutrient-dense, plant-based foods. Your body and mind will be so happy you took the time to do this.

7

EAT Habits

We, as a country, have adopted some habits that have negatively impacted our quality of life. SAD (Standard American Diet) is one example of this. We get complacent and comfortable with the same old way of living; we settle. It's important to remember that we can rise above the mediocrity and rock our lives! We have the choice and the gift to live our best life *now*. Every moment of every day is an opportunity for a do-over, and it begins with taking an honest inventory of your current habits to determine what's working and what's not. If we can wake up, reclaim our true selves, and start anew, then we can Thrive and shine. Let's get started with a few habits we can't wait to break.

Right Size and Right Time

A major cause of our ever-expanding waistlines and increased systemic inflammation is an epidemic of portion distortion. If we were to embrace right-size portions, we would be in a lot better shape; we would be a much more vital and thriving country. We are witnessing a trend of ever-increasing sizes for everything, from drink bottles, to cereal boxes, to family-size portions for one, to fast-food supersize meals costing less than the regular size. It has gotten to where we hardly know what a realistic, healthy size is anymore. What once was supersize is the new normal. The average size of a fast-food meal or order of fries has nearly quadrupled in the last thirty years.[1] As the size of our portions increase, so do we—and so do our children.

Overeating is a national problem, and it is one of the main contributing factors of obesity and being overweight. The number of obese children has skyrocketed as their self-esteem has plummeted. According to the Obesity Society, obesity causes at least 300,000 deaths each year in the United States,[2] and the healthcare costs associated with obesity in adults (reported in 2012) is estimated at $190 billion.[3]

Give Your Diet a Hand

Here's a quick way to size up healthy eating (per meal) by using your hand as a guide:

- **Palm = Proteins:** Most protein portions should be about the size of your palm (when you cup your hand). Concentrated protein is found largely in animal products, like fish, poultry, meats, and cottage cheese. Some veggie protein sources include legumes, tofu, and tempeh.
- **Thumb = Fats:** Fats are important, but they're also very dense; so, match fat portions to the size of your thumb. Good fat sources are olive oil, coconut oil, nuts, and seeds; unsalted organic butter is also good. You can also use your thumb to measure out about an ounce of cheese. Note: Nuts and seeds vary considerably in nutrient density. While they are highly

nutritious, they are also high-calorie. Our general recommendation is about 2 tablespoons nuts or seeds (about one handful, or two shot glasses).

- **Fist = Fruits, Grains, Etc.:** Your bread, fruit, cereal, rice, and grain portions should be about equal to the size of your closed fist, or a tennis ball. Remember that it's always preferable to consume whole grains and whole fruits as opposed to processed foods, fruit juices, or fruit concentrates.
- **Hand = Veggies:** Open your hand and spread your fingers as wide as you can—that's a good vegetable portion. Raw vegetables are loaded with fiber and nutrients, and they contain very few calories.

Obesity is swiftly approaching tobacco as America's number one preventable risk for premature death. Think twice before you supersize; it may literally change the course of your life. And there are already many tools available to help you understand what a healthy portion size looks like. Using a kitchen scale is, of course, one of the most effective ways, but we know that can become burdensome and time consuming (and we're all about efficiency).

Overeating increases inflammation, as does carrying extra fat. The more calories we consume, the greater the likelihood that we will gain weight—and the more likely we will die prematurely, from diseases that could have been prevented altogether. So how do you keep from overeating, and what can you do to keep your overall caloric intake at a healthy level for your body? Besides eating right-sized portions, we recommend that you eat at regular intervals, and never let more than three hours pass between eating or snacking. We call this meal frequency (MF). Not only is this great for your metabolism but it's also great for your brain. Your brain lives on glucose, and it is feeding whether you are eating or not,

24/7. Eating every three to three and a half hours will give your brain the glucose it needs to function at its highest level.

Also, pay attention to how full you are as you eat. (There are a few ways to do all of this mindfully.) Remember the Okinawan diet? One of the important components of the Okinawan lifestyle is that people stop eating before they actually feel full. It takes our brains a little time to catch up with our bellies when it comes to registering fullness. Okinawans call this way of eating *hara hachi bu*, which translates to "eat until you are 80 percent full." This philosophy is so simple yet so profound.

Another effective strategy for managing portions, timing, and overall food intake is what is referred to as the Hunger Scale. There are many diet programs that successfully use this strategy as a way of determining where your true level of hunger lies. The Hunger Scale is basically a tool where you rate your degree of hunger from 1 to 10—where 1 is actually starving to the point of weakness, possible headache, mental confusion or fogginess, and shakiness; and 10 is feeling so full you can hardly move, you are physically uncomfortable, and you don't even want to think about food. The ideal time to eat is when you are between a 3 and 6 on the Hunger Scale: at 3, you have a strong desire to eat and feel noticeably hungry; and at 6, you are fairly satisfied but could use a small snack (preferably under 300 calories).

When you allow yourself to get below a 3, you set yourself up for blood sugar fluctuations, and the body starts to hold on to fat because it thinks it's getting ready to go into starvation mode. Chances are that when you get around food (think about not eating all day, driving home in traffic, and coming home to a pantry full of chips and cookies), you are going to stuff your face with anything and everything that is readily available. This is not an optimal situation when you are working on portion control. Similarly, if you are at a 7 or 8, your coworker just swung by the donut shop, and you decide to indulge (even though you're not hungry), you are most likely setting yourself up for indigestion, discomfort, and weight gain.

Author Check-In

Debra's mindful eating: James has always had a healthy appetite—and by "healthy," I mean robust. Early in our relationship, it was so exciting to cook together and eat together that I was eating almost as much as he was. Having seconds was the norm. And I was having so much fun with the newness of the relationship that it took many months to learn that not only did I not need to keep up with his calorie intake, if I did, I was going to gain a lot of weight. I didn't like feeling so full either. It was empowering to recognize the behavior and be able to turn it around.

Fast-forward more than twenty years later, and even James has transformed his way of eating by bringing mindfulness to the table with every meal. We've altered our portions considerably, for example. In past years, we may have each had a chicken breast at dinner (6 to 8 ounces); and now, if we do have chicken, we'll usually split one breast for two or three of us (3 to 4 ounces). We have become especially mindful of animal-based portions as well as grains; and we stick to a plant-based diet.

•   •   •   •   •   •   •   •   •   •   •   •

ACTION STEP

Mindfulness comes through practices like *hara hachi bu* and the Hunger Scale. To do this:

- Get in touch with your stomach. Use the 80-percent-full rule and the Hunger Scale.
- Before your next meal, take a minute to breathe. Notice your body and rate your hunger from 1 to 10. Where's your hunger level at this moment? Have you allowed yourself to get overly hungry, or are you not truly hungry yet?

- Take time to breathe before and after each bite. Put your utensil down after every bite and chew thoroughly before swallowing. Take a breath and then have your next bite. It may feel slightly tedious at first, but the payoff of being more mindful of your eating will be huge. So be patient and slow it down.
- When you are eating your meal (or snack), take momentary pauses before you reach the halfway mark of finishing what's on your plate, to sense how full you feel. Are you close to 80 percent full? Listen to your mind, body, and of course, your stomach—as funny as this might sound. Begin a new dialogue of communication with your stomach so a trusting relationship can blossom.
- Be compassionate and patient with yourself as you practice these mindful techniques and learn new habits.

· · · · · · · · · · · · ·

Dr. James on the Hunger Scale
http://youtu.be/anAauNr2-bA

Breakfast Is Non-Negotiable

The National Weight Control Registry (NWCR) is a community that studies the habits of people who have enjoyed successful, long-term weight loss. It looks at everything from what, how much, and how often people are eating; and it examines exercise trends, sleep, and stress, and how these factors contribute to successful weight management. When the NWCR evaluated the habits of individuals who had lost and maintained thirty or more pounds for longer than ten years, it found that, aside from exercise, eating breakfast offered the greatest and most powerful long-lasting support.[4]

Breakfast is a metabolic game changer. When you *break* your *fast* each morning, you send a direct message to your brain to set the metabolic, fat-burning, energy-giving machine in motion. But breakfast isn't just for people looking to lose weight. Breakfast eaters enjoy many cool perks beyond the scale: greater productivity; decreased risk for depression, heart disease, and type 2 diabetes; improved self-confidence; and stronger stress resilience, cognitive health, and overall positivity. Breakfast cannot be optional or based on whether or not you have the time for it. We need to step up and own breakfast, making it an enjoyable, unshakable ritual. Use your *why* to make it happen.

Owning breakfast does not mean starting the day with sugar. Unfortunately, many of the food products labeled "breakfast food" have more sugar than a Snickers bar. And if you're a cereal eater, you've got to be especially mindful of reading ingredients lists. There are very few cereals out there that would qualify as a great breakfast choice. However, if you are wedded to the cereal ritual, here are some guidelines:

- Choose cereals made with certified non-GMO or organic whole grains.
- Try to avoid corn-based cereals or corn-sweetened cereals. Basically, if corn is on the label, put it back on the shelf. Why? Genetically modified (GM) corn is littered throughout our food supply. Unless it is labeled organic corn, chances are it is genetically modified. Genetically modified foods can contribute to an increasing number of health concerns, including reproductive, digestive, and hormonal challenges.[5]
- Choose cereals with a minimum of 5 grams of fiber.
- Choose cereals with at least 8 grams of protein, preferably 10.
- Choose cereals that do not contain high-fructose corn syrup, partially hydrogenated oils, food coloring, and artificial flavoring.

Over half the cereals on supermarket shelves are made up of 24 to 26 percent sugar by weight. The Environmental Working Group looked into this and found that one of the worst offenders, Kellogg's Honey Smacks, weighing in at over 50 percent sugar, had a greater percentage of sugar in one serving than a Twinkie.[6]

We have better ideas for breakfast, many of which you'll find in the 30-day TEMT meal plan. Some of our favorite breakfasts:

- Greek yogurt with a half-cup of berries, and a sprinkling of ground flax and walnuts
- A poached egg over sautéed spinach, with an avocado quarter
- A protein smoothie made with almond milk, whey protein, and fresh supergreens (baby spinach, kale, parsley, chard, etc.)
- Gluten-free or grain-free pancakes or muffins balanced by some healthy lean protein and/or whey protein (or sprouted brown-rice protein) added to the batter (This one is better on weekends, when you have a bit more time to splurge. We'll share a few of these recipes in the meal plan section of the book.)

• • • • • • • • • • • •

ACTION STEP

Make a commitment right now to add breakfast to your schedule this week, and journal about how it feels when you follow through (or don't) every day. Even if you already eat breakfast, commit to one of the TEMT breakfast options each day (no sugary cereals or fast-food breakfasts of convenience); then write down how it feels right after you eat and halfway through your morning. Even just a few words (like *wonderful* or *focused*—we're hoping for words like this, at least!) will help show you how making breakfast a habit will help you Thrive every day.

• • • • • • • • • • • •

Dr. James on Breakfast
http://www.youtube.com/watch?v=pZSZS0INy6Y&list=PLDF2
6DC5254801299

Feed Your Muscles

We often have people ask us about what and when to eat after a workout. Crushing your post-workout recovery meal will serve you long after the sweat has dried. The right foods and right timing burn extra fat, keep your metabolism moving for hours, and support you in having the energy and stamina to want to do it again the next day with zeal and passion.

With every workout and exercise bout, our bodies use fuel in the form of glycogen to support the energy needs of our muscles. When you push your body to the limit, your muscles will be nearly or fully depleted of it. Glycogen is responsible for enabling our muscles to work, run, stretch, lift, and perform. From the time you are finished exercising until roughly thirty to forty-five minutes later, your muscles and body are in what is referred to as a "glycogen window." Feed your muscles the right food during a glycogen window and your body responds in kind, refueling the muscle energy tank, repairing broken-down muscle tissue, and driving fat-burning metabolism for hours after your workout.

This simple and powerful practice can be a game changer. When we miss the glycogen window and choose not to eat, guess what? We increase inflammation, discourage optimum fat burning, and set ourselves up for a poorer performance with our next workout.

The optimal foods to fuel recovery on all levels are a combination of easily digestible proteins and readily absorbed carbohydrates. Aim for 15 to 20 grams of protein after each workout. Strong research suggests that whey protein (as well as sprouted plant-based proteins) is an awesome choice to ensure superior and efficient digestibility. Whey protein contains a powerful array of amino acids (important energy sources for muscle) and branched-chain amino acids—essential nutrients that assist muscle repair and muscle building, prevent fatigue, and improve resilience under stress. Carbohydrates should come from organic whole grains, vegetables, and fruit to replace the lost glycogen and maximize amino-acid synthesis. This process is instrumental in "driving" the protein into the muscle cell for optimal benefit. And this eating strategy is easily incorporated after each and every workout by having a whey-protein-based smoothie with fresh berries. The key is to plan ahead, remembering that once you are finished with your sweat session, the clock is ticking. So, refuel your way to optimum wellness and thriving.

The Dirty Dozen and the Clean Fifteen

Every year, the Environmental Working Group (www.ewg.org) puts out a shopper's guide to pesticide residue levels in foods. In their guide, they refer to the "Dirty Dozen," a list of the twelve fruits and vegetables with the highest levels of pesticides, as well as the "Clean Fifteen," a list of produce with the lowest measured levels. Here is a summary of their findings from 2013.

Dirty Dozen:

Apples	Imported nectarines
Celery	Peaches
Cherry tomatoes	Potatoes
Cucumbers	Spinach
Grapes	Strawberries
Hot peppers (like jalapeños)	Bell peppers

The Clean Fifteen:

Asparagus	Mangoes
Avocados	Mushrooms
Cabbages	Onions
Cantaloupes	Papayas
Corn	Pineapples
Eggplants	Frozen sweet peas
Grapefruits	Sweet potatoes
Kiwis	

Do what you can to choose organic produce whenever possible. And if organic isn't an option, aim for foods on the Clean Fifteen list. Note that this list can change from year to year. You can stay updated by visiting the Environmental Working Group online: ewg.org/foodnews/index.php.

Fighting Fire with Fiber

A very important component of TEMT is hearty fiber intake. Fiber serves up so much good, yet it gets so little respect. One of the few things proven to help keep hunger pangs at bay, keep you feeling satiated longer, and support a healthy digestive tract is fiber. Getting your daily fill of fiber will move your life from average to amazing in both mind and body.

One of the primary causes of inflammation is the spiking of blood sugar and insulin due to the ingestion of highly processed and refined junk foods devoid of fiber. When we eat fiber-free foods, we create an environment ripe for systemic inflammation.

Chronic inflammation spikes can damage the brain over time by allowing toxins to seep into brain cells. If you have ever been on a junk-food binge and felt that hazy, lazy, slow way of being, you have been under the influence of these toxins.

Many of the popular diets that Americans tend to gravitate toward are extremely low in fiber. Most of the high-protein diets that encourage high protein and low to no carbs, have barely—if any—mention of fiber. This approach to dieting will not only tax your colon, heart, and kidneys, but it will also challenge your digestion and support systemic inflammation, not to mention constipation.

Most prepackaged diet foods, junk foods, and even popular breakfast foods are fiber deficient. This includes cereal, of course. When we begin the day with this type of fiber-deficient cereal and milk—the way

Top Ten Fiber-Rich Foods

1. Beans and legumes: black beans, pinto beans, white beans, lentils
2. Flaxseeds, sesame seeds, sunflower seeds (raw, not roasted and salted), chia seeds, hemp seeds
3. Kale, broccoli, spinach, Brussels sprouts
4. Sweet potatoes
5. Quinoa
6. Almonds, pistachios, pecans, walnuts
7. Berries, cherries
8. Artichokes, carrots, celery
9. Avocados
10. Kiwis, pears, oranges, apples

many of the school-age children in our country do—we set ourselves up for a spike in blood sugar followed by a rapid fall, an increased craving for more junk food throughout the day, and a major energy drain.

C-reactive protein (CRP) is an inflammatory messenger, and when CRP levels are higher than normal, there is an increased risk for heart disease, stroke, and having a heart attack. Fiber can lower CRP.[7] And the more fiber we eat, the lower our risk for systemic inflammation.

Increasing our fiber intake delivers significant results. Data from the Nurses' Health Studies revealed that women reduce their risk for heart disease by 20 percent for each ten grams of fiber consumed.[8] Multiply that by three (as in 30 grams of fiber/day) and you're cutting your risk by 60 percent!

When our diets become more plant-based, we significantly lower our risk of cardiovascular disease and stroke.[9] The nutrients found in a plant-based diet contain antioxidants, omega-3 fatty acids, mono- and polyunsaturated fatty acids, phytochemicals, and fiber—all of which help lower systemic inflammation.

Setting any intention, such as meeting your daily fiber needs (for men, it is 38 grams; for women, 25 grams), will ultimately support sustained energy, healthier digestion, and a more balanced and steady mood and focus. Improved cholesterol ratios, insulin sensitivity, and overall improved heart health may go unnoticed at first, but underneath it all, your body will reap the benefits of decreased inflammation.

• • • • • • • • • • • •

ACTION STEP

To work toward a habit of getting enough fiber, set the intention of doing so for at least one week. See how you feel and how easily you can incorporate higher fiber options into your daily routine. Some ideas are:

- At breakfast, set a goal of getting at least 10 grams of fiber—easily accomplished with high-fiber cereals and a serving of ground flax, nuts, and berries; whole-grain toast with a serving of almond butter; or a protein smoothie with berries and ground flaxseeds, chia seeds, or hemp seeds.
- Follow that morning fiber hit with a midmorning snack: a handful of almonds or an apple with almond butter.
- For lunch, aim for another 10 grams of fiber. This is done easily by choosing whole-grain bread as the base for your sandwich; bean or lentil soup; a piece of fruit; a hearty salad, plus a sprinkle of seeds.
- Add fiber to your midafternoon snack with sliced veggies, hummus, flax-based crackers, a serving of nuts or seeds, or a fiber-enhanced smoothie.
- Finish fiber-strong at dinner by opting for a veggie-rich stir-fry over a bed of quinoa or brown rice, kale salad with a lean protein, or a veggie-/bean-based soup.

• • • • • • • • • • • •

Fiber is key to overall nutrition and healthy weight management. Most fiber-rich foods have a low glycemic index value (meaning they help glucose release more slowly into the bloodstream) and play a vital role in helping slow down the rate at which sugar enters the bloodstream.

Fiber-rich foods are more satisfying because they help the body register a feeling of fullness. When you eat foods rich in fiber, satiety—that feeling of being satisfied after a meal—happens sooner and lasts longer compared to when you eat refined, fiberless foods.

There are basically two types of fiber: soluble and insoluble. Both are essential for good health and optimal digestion. Once in the body and absorbed, soluble fiber forms a sticky gel that acts like a protective coating, preventing harmful substances from doing damage in the gut. One study showed that when we include at least 7 grams of soluble fiber daily, it significantly decreases the risk of dying from heart disease.[10] Great soluble fiber sources include prunes, avocados, black beans, artichokes, sweet potatoes, dates, figs, and apples.

Insoluble fiber is a type of fiber that comes from the structural material of plants. It stimulates movement in the intestinal tract and dilutes the concentration of toxins that may be residing in the colon. Sources of insoluble fiber include avocados, blackberries, guava, wheat bran, lentils, broccoli, Brussels sprouts, mung beans, and carrots.

More Fiber—Plus Water

When it comes to fiber, one other thing that's important to remember is water. Water hydrates and lubricates our tissues and joints; helps eliminate wastes and toxins from our tissues; and is crucial in our body's ability to transport vital nutrients, proteins, sugars, electrolytes, minerals, and vitamins throughout the body for proper assimilation. You should always try to drink half your weight (in ounces) of water; and when you increase the amount of fiber in your diet, you need to increase your intake of water too. This is because fiber acts sort of like a sponge in your system: it soaks up fluids, increasing the need to adequately hydrate all the cells of your body so they can do their best work. Making sure the fiber remains well lubricated and slippery allows it to pass entirely through your system, grabbing debris along the way, and not getting stuck somewhere in your intestines.

Some fabulous ways to get fiber:

Source	Total Fiber
½ cup broccoli florets	4 to 5 grams
½ cup beans	6 to 10 grams
3 figs	10 grams
½ cup kale or spinach	4 to 6 grams
½ cup berries	5 grams
¼ cup almonds	3 grams

Exercise: One Meal at a Time

This is your opportunity to improve your life by implementing a few of the practices we have mentioned. Begin today with breakfast (remember, it's non-negotiable), and practice portion control right off the bat. Consider having just one egg, one piece of whole-grain toast (or one gluten-free waffle), and half a grapefruit. Choose just one cup of coffee—and skip the sugar.

Practice *hara hachi bu* at every meal. Create a little sign as a reminder, and place it on the dining room table or refrigerator. Keep a reminder on your desk at work, and keep a sticky note in your car if you tend to make a habit of eating there (we don't recommend this, by the way.) Make note of where you can sneak in additional fiber during the day. Add ground flax to your morning yogurt, oatmeal, or smoothie, or sprinkle it on your lunch greens. Snack on fresh vegetables, nuts, and seeds. Choose whole grains over processed white-flour based products. Become a fiber fanatic. And between snacks and meals, drink plenty of water—at least eight glasses per day, adding a few more if you work out regularly and even more if you sweat a lot during exercise.

8

EAT for Your Brain

While we often think of our bodies—or at least, what our bodies look like—when it comes to what we put in our mouths, we sometimes forget about the brain–food connection. This connection affects not just how we feel, but also how we continue to eat as our lives progress.

As we discussed in THINK, your inner pharmacy of neurotransmitters are fed, built, and sustained by the foods you choose to eat. You have both the opportunity and the responsibility to feed your brain well. When your brain is well nourished, it is capable of producing genius thoughts, creativity, positivity, and loving emotions, along with peace and calm. Take a moment to consider how your life would be impacted by knowing—deeply trusting—that you have the tools and the power to feel good and be at your best every day.

Growing Your Brain

There are important ways to feed your brain—positive ways. When fed foods that contain the right chemical compounds, the brain can actually grow. One of these compounds is a powerful protein called *brain-derived neurotrophic factor* (BDNF). (Some scientists refer to this protein as Miracle-Gro for the brain.) BDNF supports the brain by encouraging the growth of nerve cells and synapses, which translates to improved cognition, long-term memory, and other positive mental and emotional traits—this is what we mean by growing your brain. It's the building of new nerve cells and connections that in turn grows our brilliance. Whether you are nine years old or ninety, you can put BDNF to work for you. Dark-green leafy vegetables; deep-sea, cold-water fish like salmon, halibut, cod, sardines (rich in omega-3 fatty acids); nuts; and seeds are all building blocks that feed and grow BDNF. And as you improve the status of BDNF in your brain, the areas that are responsible for thinking clearly and positively, and supporting healthy memory, are fed to become more vital.

Top Ten Daily Focus Foods (Foods that Serve the Brain)

Fish
Nuts
Blueberries (berries are great in general)
Apples
Red onions
Rosemary
Flaxseeds
Olive oil
Dark, leafy greens
Cherries

Wondering what may negatively affect BDNF? Stress, saturated fat, alcohol, excess sugar, and other aspects of SAD (Standard American

Diet) will decrease levels of BDNF.[1] When BDNF decreases, our risk of depression, memory challenges, and brain atrophy (shrinking) increases.

 Making BDNF Work for You
http://www.youtube.com/watch?v=CdTKxHhHZ1I&list=PLDF2 6DC5254801299

De-Stress Through Diet

A 2007 poll conducted by the American Psychological Association found that one-third of Americans report experiencing extreme levels of stress. About one in five said they have high levels of stress fifteen or more days per month.[2] Being "too busy" is one of the primary reasons we don't deal with stress, yet there are simple and effective ways to de-stress your life through prudent and empowering dietary choices.

Chronic, uncontrolled stress drives our cravings for sugar and other less-than-awesome foods and beverages. When you increase or abuse stimulants (such as caffeine), you add insult to injury. Having a daily cup or two of organic coffee or tea is fine; they both contain robust antioxidants. But when you overdo the brew, too much caffeine can send an already overtaxed, overcharged, and overstimulated nervous system into overdrive. When this happens, your adrenal glands respond by producing excessive levels of the stress hormone cortisol.

We touched on cortisol in the THINK section but want to talk about it now in relation to why, how, and what we eat. SAD has impaired the work of cortisol in the body. Sugar, fruit juice, and overly processed foods release sugar into the bloodstream rapidly, which negatively impacts cortisol and insulin. Chronically high cortisol is a surefire way to put yourself on the fast track to gaining fat, losing vitality, and increasing your risk for type 2 diabetes and heart disease, not to mention a whole host of other chronic yet preventable diseases.

Some Dietary Antistress Measures

- Decrease consumption of caffeinated beverages like soda, coffee, and energy drinks (weakens adrenals / adrenal response to stress)
- Decrease alcohol
- Decrease refined carbohydrates (chips, cookies, muffins, crackers, cakes)
- Increase complex carbohydrates (Here's your list: greens [spinach, kale, watercress, lettuce, mustard greens, Swiss chard, broccoli], most fruits and vegetables, most whole grains [whole barley, buckwheat, oat bran, spelt, oats, brown rice, wild rice], yogurt, legumes [lentils, garbanzos, soy beans, black beans, pinto beans], onions, tomatoes)

High levels of cortisol trigger the release of a whole army of physiological players associated with stress. One of these players is the hormone leptin, which tells us when we are full. Leptin is actually produced in our adipose (fat) tissue. When we become chronically stressed, we tend to become less sensitive to leptin; as a consequence, we overeat. Reason may tell us that more leptin would result in fewer cravings, but since it is produced in fat tissue, obese individuals often have too much of it. This actually compromises leptin function (much like a bottleneck traffic jam), and leptin resistance becomes an issue. The result is having out-of-control sugar cravings and an inability to know when you are really full. The solution is TEMT: whole foods, stress reduction, meal planning, portion control, and exercise.

Stress can also have an opposite effect on appetite. Some people lose their appetite under stress, and fail to consume adequate calories and nutrients. This sets them up for nutrient deficiencies and puts them at risk for many health challenges.

Chronic stress and high cortisol have a direct effect on mood and optimism. Excess cortisol in the body shuts down serotonin; and when serotonin drops, risk of depression increases. High cortisol and excess stress also shut down the hormone melatonin. This may explain why we don't sleep well when we're under a lot of stress or when we overdo it with sugar. This lack of sleep prevents us from making GH (growth hormone—remember from the THINK section?), which is produced mainly while we are engaged in deep sleep.

Sugar and stress place excess pressure on our adrenal glands, and this makes us feel exhausted all the time, putting us at risk for anxiety. We tend to want to feed our emotions, and we crave comfort foods in the form of refined sugar and carbs (to boost serotonin). This vicious cycle leaves us unsatisfied, unhappy, and overweight. But when we follow through on meal frequency, portion control, and adequate fiber consumption, we are more likely to healthfully navigate our cravings.

Targeting and Preventing Stress with Herbs

- St. John's wort eases mild depression caused by stress.
- Rhodiola (aka rosenroot or golden root) is one of our favorite herbs when we are feeling a bit run down. It reduces stress, burnout, and anxiety; and it may lower cortisol.[3]
- Siberian ginseng and Panax ginseng strengthen and tonify the adrenal glands.
- Other herbs that are wonderful as a tea include passionflower, chamomile, and valerian root. [Debra: sipping chamomile tea about a half hour before bed is a nice and calming ritual.]
- If you're unable to fall asleep, consider supplementing melatonin (3 milligrams thirty minutes prior to going to bed).

The TEMT approach to eating is spot-on for keeping cortisol and other hormones in balance. Meal frequency supports healthy and balanced blood sugar levels. TEMT foods also fight stress and cortisol by supporting a healthy balance of macronutrients: carbohydrates, proteins, and fats. Help your body fight back against stress by feeding your cells a wide variety of phytonutrients: include a generous mix of vegetables and fresh fruit.

Under stress, the body can lose valuable stores of vitamins, minerals, amino acids, and other important nutrients. Certain foods rich in these nutrients may help to keep your system strong under stress and possibly offset the damage stress causes. Your ability to handle stress is largely dependent on antioxidants, including vitamins C and E; B vitamins, which prevent fatigue and are vital to immunity and nerve-cell activity; and magnesium, which helps prevent depression and relieve muscle tension. (On a side note, nutritional deficiencies can show up in a number of ways, so we suggest a daily multivitamin as one part of your preventive strategy.)

When we are under stress, the body begins to produce free radicals, increasing inflammation in the body and taking down the immune system. As an antioxidant, vitamin C fights against free-radical damage and supports healthy immunity. And vitamin C is essential for efficient adrenal gland performance—another way it helps us manage stress. Foods highest in vitamin C include strawberries, bell peppers, oranges and other citrus fruits, kiwi, broccoli, kale and other dark-green leafy vegetables, and guavas.

B vitamins may have the best known reputation as antistress vitamins. Chronic stress and poor lifestyle choices (bad diet, lack of quality sleep, lack of exercise, and so on) can drain the body of B vitamins. B5 (pantothenic acid) and B6 (pyridoxine) support adrenal health, so when stress puts the adrenals on overdrive, these vitamins are comprised. B vitamins also support a healthy nervous system. Under stress, the nervous system shifts into "fight or flight" mode and the body calls in extra nutrients to help calm the storm. Like vitamin C, the B vitamins are water-soluble—the body does not store them. We need to continuously consume foods high in these vitamins or consider supplementing. Some foods rich in B vitamins: bananas, broccoli, eggs, fish, kale, milk, nuts, spinach, whole grains.

Omega-3 fatty acids challenge stress by helping to lower systemic inflammation and supporting healthy immunity. Deep-sea, cold-water fish are great sources of omega-3s. Vegetarian sources of omega-3 fatty acids include flaxseed, chia, hemp, walnuts, avocados, and Brussels sprouts. If you are not eating many foods from this list and are vegan, you may consider vegetarian-sourced omega-3 supplements.

Chronic stress can deplete the body's magnesium, and magnesium plays a vital role in healthy adrenal function, immunity, heart health, the nervous system, and overall energy. Sources of magnesium include pumpkin seeds, halibut, black beans, sesame seeds, cashews, spinach, kale, almonds, sunflower seeds, chard, Brazil nuts, avocados, yogurt, and dark chocolate.

Zinc levels also decrease under stress, but you can combat this through food sources like crab, oysters, pork, poultry, beans, cashews, and yogurt.

Under stress, our brain uses serotonin. When our stores of serotonin become low due to stress (extended stress), our mood is compromised and the risk for anxiety and depression increases. Fortunately, complex carbohydrates can help to raise serotonin levels (quinoa, dark green leafy vegetables, brown rice, sprouted wheat). Eating fewer simple carbohydrates also helps, so avoid refined sugar; corn syrup; fruit juice; candy; cake, bread, pasta, and any other foods made with white flour; soda (carbonated beverages); and most packaged cereals. These foods only increase the negative impact of stress on the body.

It is equally important to avoid missing meals, as this can lead to blood sugar fluctuations and cause moodiness, weakness, weight gain, brain fog, and an increased risk for type 2 diabetes.

Stress-Busting Foods

- Foods rich in vitamin C: oranges, mangoes, guava, bell peppers, watermelons, lemons, papayas, grapefruits, kiwis, broccoli, Brussels sprouts, cauliflower, strawberries, tomatoes, kale, cabbage
- Foods rich in vitamin B5: turkey (dark meat), brewer's yeast, peanuts, chicken (dark meat), eggs, brown rice, sweet corn, lean beef, sweet potatoes, cashews, soy
- Foods rich in vitamin B6: watermelons, bananas, salmon, avocados, turkey and chicken, rainbow trout, tomatoes, sunflower seeds, soy, halibut, sweet potatoes, oats, tuna, brown rice, broccoli, beef, garbanzo beans, pineapples, walnuts, brewer's yeast, hazelnuts
- Carbohydrates that raise serotonin levels (by raising tryptophan levels): oatmeal, peanuts, granola, raisins, wheat germ, collard greens, whole wheat, sweet potatoes, yogurt, spinach
- Foods rich in zinc: oysters, toasted wheat germ, turkey, cheese, Swiss chard, beef, pumpkin seeds, mustard greens, soy, tuna, baked potatoes, lima beans, ginger root, rice, lentils, leeks, sunflower seeds, cashews, pecans, nuts, whole grains
- Foods rich in potassium: avocados, apricots, potatoes, cantaloupes, lima beans, parsnips, raisins, sardines, soy, broccoli, tomatoes, legumes, bananas, milk, sweet potatoes, salmon, peaches, spinach, mustard greens, turkey, celery, tuna, peanuts, papayas, asparagus, apples, cauliflower
- Foods rich in magnesium: acorn squash, dates, artichokes, raisins, avocados, spinach, butternut squash, watermelons, figs, dairy products, meat, seafood, bananas, black-eyed peas, blueberries, chickpeas, kidney beans, lentils, navy beans, pinto beans, potatoes, rice, sesame seeds, spinach, split peas, zucchini

Dr. James on Magnesium
http://www.youtube.com/watch?v=7SMngZZ7C4U&list=PLDF2
6DC5254801299

Cravings Disarmed

Think of the last time that you had an uncontrollable craving. Was it during your commute home and you hadn't had anything to eat in several hours? When you finally made it home, were you famished? What were you craving—broccoli or kale? We're guessing not. Most likely, you wanted cake, cookies, Chardonnay (or insert your nonwater beverage of choice here), or all of the above.

This insatiable craving for sugar and other refined carbohydrates is your brain and body doing what it needs to do to reestablish serotonin levels as fast as possible. Sugar is a quick fix, but it will not sustain you or your mood; you will be left looking for more sugar to fill the craving. To help you navigate stress, keep your serotonin strong. It will help you to keep it all together—mood, food, and outlook—by taking an offensive stance rather than a defensive one, crushing cravings and boosting your mood.

Too often we lean on willpower to help us overcome our cravings, but willpower is only as strong as your balanced blood sugar.

• • • • • • • • • • • •

ACTION STEP

- Fill your fridge and pantry with healthy snacks. This seems obvious, but most of us keep a few stashes of sweet and/or salty junk foods around the house, thinking we've got our cravings under control. Remember, most cravings are emotionally driven and will subside in twenty minutes or less.

- Bait and switch your cravings by giving yourself something better. Nighttime cravings are made less attractive when you choose instead to take a bubble bath, chat with a loved one, or curl up with a good book or movie.
- Keep a snack-attack journal and notice when you get the hunger pangs for sweets. Is it a certain time of the day, a certain action that triggers the craving, or a certain person who makes you want to eat something less than healthy? Once you identify the trigger, you can work to release it.
- Keep a stash of nuts and/or seeds in your desk at work, your purse, and/or your car so you can fuel yourself with some good nutrition before you find yourself running on empty.
- Remember to stay hydrated. Sometimes thirst and dehydration mimic hunger.

• • • • • • • • • • • •

Author Check-In

Debra's craving busters: I notice that when I step into the natural food store and I'm moderately hungry, I want something immediately. It could be that the store itself triggers a craving. In the past, I was drawn to grabbing a baked good like a scone, muffin, or cookie; but I never felt energized after indulging in the craving. The same was true when I indulged in kettle corn at the farmer's market; I loved the crunch but didn't love how I felt after a few handfuls. What really works for me is to have something crunchy on hand. Raw almonds or macadamia nuts are my favorite craving busters. If I'm craving something sweet and crunchy, then I will have an apple. Nuts, seeds, or a fresh piece of fruit are really satisfying to me and help sustain my energy until I have time for a real meal.

Food for Thought

As we now know, the foods we eat are directly linked to the hormones, glucose, and neurotransmitters that nourish our brain. When you follow a plant-based eating program like TEMT, you help protect your brain from degenerative diseases like dementia and Alzheimer's, and protect your thinking from negativity. The more plant-based your diet, the greater the protection you get from antioxidants, B vitamins, and other nutrients that support your body and your brain. When your diet is low in plant-based nutrients and high in animal-based products, you increase the rate of free-radial production and fuel the development of disease.

In support of keeping our thinking fine tuned and full of possibility, taking a proactive stance in treating our brain to the very best in loving care just makes sense. We have a powerful impact on how healthfully our brain, mind, and memory function throughout life. The lifestyle choices that we make may be the best brain and memory medicine around.

A diet rich in key nutrients are a brain's best friend. Here's what to add to your shopping cart: blueberries, broccoli, cauliflower, cabbage, Brussels sprouts, mustard greens, spinach, kale, and dark-green leafy veggies. These foods all support memory and cognition; and the leafy greens and spinach are a good source of the B vitamin folate. Folate has attracted a lot of recent attention due to its potential in protecting against cognitive decline.[4] Other folate-rich foods include beans, legumes, and fortified grains.

Deep-sea, cold-water, fatty (wild) fish is one of the best brain foods, full of anti-inflammatory omega-3 fatty acids. Adding one serving of fish per week may decrease the risk of Alzheimer's disease by nearly 60 percent.[5] Consumption of wild fish (versus farmed) supports a positive mood and optimistic outlook.

Nuts and seeds contain healthy fats plus vitamin E, which has been associated with a reduced risk of Alzheimer's disease. When cruising the snack section, reach for your favorites (think walnuts, hazelnuts, almonds, pumpkin seeds, hemp seeds).

Turmeric (aka curcumin) is another powerful force in helping lower the risk of Alzheimer's disease. Turmeric is an awesome addition to stir-fries and salad dressings, and you'll recognize it as the ingredient that typically makes most curries bright yellow.

To add to your food for thought, consider green tea. Green tea (*Camellia sinensis*) is rich in a mighty brain-protective antioxidant called epigallocatechin gallate (EGCG). Research published in the *American Journal of Clinical Nutrition* found that people who regularly drink green tea have sharper minds then those who do not drink green tea. Having as little as four to six cups per week resulted in 38 percent less cognitive impairment.[6] We can enthusiastically raise a mug and toast to that!

You have the tools that you need to Thrive; you just have to decide that you're ready—that you're worth it. Fortunately, food is simple, and for the most part, so is eating. Consider and look at your ROI—your Return on Ingestion—and invest wisely in what you want. Decide what outcome you are looking for, and build your diet and your life based on that vision.

Now that you know how food can shift your mind and your thinking, it's up to you to choose wisely. Food is first about nourishment. After that, it is up to you to decide how you use food. What you put in your mouth has to do with how you want to show up and perform in this life. We want you to show up big. We want you to Thrive.

Exercise: Grow Your Brain

Remember, BDNF (brain-derived neurotrophic factor) protein is a catalyst that helps improve brain function. Here are three things you can do today to raise your BDNF, improve mental clarity, and decrease your risk for depression and Alzheimer's disease:

1. Keep your blood sugar balanced with meal frequency.
2. Snack on ¼ cup of walnuts.
3. Serve up a curry dish for dinner.

EAT

Summary

Eat with intention.

- Focus on your primary "foods" (things that feed your soul)—your relationships, your career, your community—to build a foundation for the rest of your life.
- Set an intention every morning to be present to your highest potential, and then make food choices that support this.
- Discover your eating personality so you know what psychological state you start from when eating.
- Consider how to best alter or support your eating personality for living your highest potential.

Inflammation is a widespread epidemic that can often be prevented through diet.

- SAD (Standard American Diet) feeds the fire of inflammation; TEMT cools it down.

133

- Think plant-based and nutrient-dense eating: the traditional Okinawan, Mediterranean, and anti-inflammatory diets are good places to start.
- Consider periodic cleansing with the changing of the seasons, or at least a few times a year.
- Simple lifestyle shifts can decrease exposure to toxins and buildup of toxicity, naturally keeping your body in balance.

Look at the habits that affect your eating. Change the ones that need to be changed and adopt new ones that will support your highest self.

- Embrace portions that are right-sized, not the oversized portions of SAD.
- Practice *hara hachi bu*—eating until you are just 80 percent full.
- Eat breakfast every day.
- Eat a high-protein snack after every workout.
- Focus on high-fiber foods.

Feed your brain the foods it needs.

- Eat foods that support BDNF to help your brain grow.
- Acknowledge how stress impacts your eating choices (comfort foods or fasting are the two most common inclinations). Infuse your diet with the foods, vitamins, and minerals it needs to deal with stress in a healthy way.
- Take an offensive stance with cravings by eating to keep your serotonin levels high.
- Eat to protect your brain from degenerative diseases like Alzheimer's and dementia by eating to decrease free-radical production.

Part III

MOVE

PART III: MOVE

> Lack of activity destroys the good condition of every
> human being, while movement and methodical physical
> exercise save it and preserve it.
>
> **—Plato**

Exercise strengthens the heart and bones; increases the effectiveness and strength of the immune system; reduces the risk for type 2 diabetes and heart disease; and optimizes metabolism. Vigorous exercise will enhance your mood, make you more productive, increase your IQ, improve your sex drive, strengthen your confidence and self-esteem, and allow your mind to flourish. Exercise will also reduce your risk for cancer; improve your sleep; help control your weight; and help protect your bones, muscles, and vital organs. Now, if we all know that, why don't we move our bodies every day?

According to statistics from the CDC (Centers for Disease Control), fewer than half of all adults meet the national guidelines for physical activity (150 minutes per week), and fewer than 30 percent of high school students get sixty minutes of physical activity every day.[1] Physical inactivity is actually a leading cause of death in this country, second only to tobacco use.[2] Moving is an absolute must in your daily practice of living, and it will change your life in the best way. Are you open and willing to commit to moving daily—as if your very life depended on it?

Adults must make time to exercise every day, with an ideal goal of about 150 minutes a week (equivalent to thirty minutes, five times per week). The activity should be demanding enough to make you breathe harder, feel warmer, and sweat a little (or a lot). And of course, kids need exercise too. The goal for children is to get an hour of exercise every day. And this doesn't have to be done all at once, by the way. Kids and adults can break up activities into several ten- or fifteen-minute segments.

Even individuals who don't begin to get active until later in life still benefit greatly from exercise once they start. A recent study published in the *British Journal of Sports Medicine* tracked the health of 3,500 men and women in the midfifties-to-midseventies age range over a period of eight years. Participants in this study were ranked in terms of health, with the top 19 percent being classified as "healthy agers." It may come as no surprise that the adults who had maintained a healthy lifestyle and exercised long before the beginning of the study landed in the group of healthy agers. You may be surprised to learn, however, that even those who didn't start exercising until later in life were three times more likely than their sedentary counterparts to land in that top 19 percent of healthy agers. The men and women who remained active throughout the eight-year study were seven times more likely to be classified in the healthy-ager group.[3] We know which group we would want to be a part of; how about you?

When we add exercise to our lives, we increase the likelihood of living longer and being stronger. Sedentary people have an increased incidence of dying from cardiovascular disease.[4] Being consistent with a vigorous exercise program increases healthy HDL cholesterol, lowers blood pressure, and increases insulin sensitivity—all of which lower your risk for cardiovascular disease.[5]

Let's face it: none of us want to admit to being sedentary or lazy, but with the stats on health in this country being what they are, many of us are. So, why is this the case, when we know exercise is good for us?

As you'll recall, *why* is a powerful question: *Why* should you exercise? *What* or *who* motivates you? *Why* do you want to feel better, look better, live longer? You may have many *whys*, and that's awesome. Perhaps you just have one. Whatever the case, use your *why* to get motivated. And if you find yourself truly questioning why you should exercise, consider joining a team or signing up for an organized walk or run that raises funds for a cause you are passionate about. And if all else fails, exercise because you can; plain and simple.

Think about how your healthy, strong body will help you complete meaningful goals. Think about why and how your commitment to being healthy and strong will inspire those you love. When you let go of fear and apprehension, and take a stand for your bigger mission and vision, you will be supported to rock each and every workout with passion and purpose. Movement raises and strengthens every area of your life.

 Dr. James on MOVE
http://youtu.be/2oAN9eoUouU

9

MOVE Your Perspective

Developing a positive body image is an essential part of optimum wellness and Thriving, and it isn't easy these days. Historically, it has been challenging for many people—probably the majority of Americans—to live up to societal standards and what is considered to be the ideal body of the times. For example, it's difficult for women to grow up in a society that tells them their beauty is all that matters and then promotes a standard of beauty that is unachievable. But it's also difficult for men; they're told that their "masculinity" and their ability to be a "good man" rely on physical strength and appearance. We have, essentially, been bombarded from an early age with distorted images of what the ideal body looks like. So, instead of looking at the amazing things our body can do, and instead of focusing on keeping it in optimum health, we only look to our "media mirrors," which tell us whether or not we are attractive enough and ignore our health.

Distorted body image (aka body dysmorphic disorder, or BDD) drives unhealthy behaviors ranging from eating disorders to excessive exercise, increased anxiety, and depression, regardless of whether a person is of normal weight or not. This distortion can be deceptive enough that it can skew and trick our body image to the degree that underweight or average-weight individuals may see themselves as overweight and overweight individuals may picture themselves at normal weight, perpetuating unhealthy lifestyle behaviors. The reality is that year after year, Americans continue to suffer from more and more diseases of lifestyle; and our body-image issues are a great place to start when it comes to learning how important movement is in our daily lives.

Heavy but Healthy

There's no denying that our society has a weight prejudice. During the 2012 Summer Olympics, there were snickers across the media about the bodies of some of the athletes—in particular, a few of the female athletes. Melbourne's *Herald-Sun* suggested that Leisel Jones, an amazing Australian swimmer and triple Olympic–gold medalist, didn't look as good in her swimsuit as she had in previous Olympic games. Editors even posted a poll, asking if people thought she was "fit enough" to be an Olympian, which led, of course, to tremendous backlash. Jessica Ennis, heptathlete in the 2012 Olympics (a heptathlon is a seven-part track-and-field event), was labeled "fat" by a UK athletics official. And the Brazilian women's soccer team was given this advice by Enow Ngachu, the Cameroon team's coach: "Brazil needs to improve their defensive system, and their players look a bit heavy to me—that might be a problem for them as well."[1]

The truth is, we cannot judge a person's fitness by the size of their body—and sometimes even their body mass index (BMI). Fitness trumps looks and whatever labels others might put on our physical appearance. Weight alone is a poor predictor of health. Remember, muscle weighs more than fat. Two people can weigh the same on the scale and be at completely different levels of fitness and health risk (for certain diseases). If you exercise daily but are still classified as "overweight," you are less likely to encounter heart problems compared to "normal weight" individuals (according to BMI standards) who don't exercise.

Being metabolically fit is the ultimate goal. *Metabolically fit* means that, aside from weight, a person has healthy blood sugar levels (and doesn't suffer from insulin resistance or diabetes), normal blood pressure, healthy triglyceride levels (meaning they are not elevated), and normal cholesterol levels (with higher high-density lipoprotein, or HDL). Daily exercise and consistent physical fitness pave the path to being metabolically fit.

When we talk about carrying extra fat on the body, we're sure most of you have heard the apple- and pear-shape descriptions and comparisons. Apple-shaped individuals are described as carrying extra fat around their midsection and abdominal region. Pear-shaped folks carry extra fat around their rear end and the lower half of their body. The way our fat is distributed is actually an important distinction that correlates with the health issues—like heart disease and metabolic syndrome—that tend to be associated with obesity.

Epidemiological studies (studies of diseases in large populations) indicate that pear-shaped fat distribution (described in medical literature as *gluteofemoral*, meaning butt, hips, and thighs) is linked to healthy cholesterol and blood glucose levels, and a decrease in risk for diabetes and heart disease. On the other hand, abdominal obesity (apple shaped) is associated with increased risk of metabolic syndrome, which includes insulin resistance, diabetes, and cardiovascular disease. Simply translated: gluteofemoral fat distribution may be protective, whereas abdominal fat distribution is harmful.

Abdominal fat is not just under the skin but often contains visceral fat, which is more metabolically active than the subcutaneous fat found around the behind. Visceral fat surrounds important organs like the liver, stomach, kidneys, and intestines. That is part of what makes it more of a health challenge, because it can smother the organs and affect their efficiency. Subcutaneous fat lives just below the surface of the skin and has not been linked to classic obesity-related health issues (heart disease, cancer, and metabolic syndrome), so having a little extra in the butt and thigh region is not as bad of a thing for your health.

Certainly genetics can play a role in whether or not you are apple- or pear-shaped, but regardless of genes, what is important to recognize is that all bodies are better with physical activity. Even if you are blessed with a body type that society deems attractive, you won't get healthy, you won't *Thrive*, by sitting around all day. Sedentary "normal weight" people are at increased risk for many of the same health challenges as abdominally obese individuals. Remember, we cannot judge ourselves or others based on appearance; true health resides below the surface.

Thin but Not Thriving

The exact opposite of being heavy but healthy is being thin but not Thriving. A person may appear trim on the outside and have a BMI under 25, but still carry too much visceral fat and not enough muscle. Take a look at most fashion runways and you'll see a person that embodies this issue. There is an actual medical term for this type of body: *metabolically obese normal weight* (MONW). Just like overweight individuals can be metabolically fit, skinny people can be metabolically obese. MONW individuals are actually predisposed to type 2 diabetes, high triglycerides, and premature heart disease. Regardless of whether you are normal weight, underweight, or overweight, solid aerobic fitness, strength training, and fitness in general are essential for reducing the risks of cardiovascular mortality, inflammation, and improving overall quality of life.

Many people—women in particular—may covet an incredibly thin body type because this correlates to society's standards of being attractive, but thin on the outside and obese on the inside is not a desirable trait. Trust us.

Up until our early twenties, many of us don't pay much attention to the actual relationship between health and the shape of the body. As long as we look good, that's all that seems to matter. As we age, beginning around our thirties and forties, we start to lose muscle—approximately a quarter of a pound a year. To protect muscle mass and strength, you need to engage in regular strength training (resistance or weight training), at least twice a week. Lean muscle mass is one of the most important components of healthy aging. An overall weakening of the body caused by a change in body composition, with a loss of muscle mass, is called *sarcopenia*. Too little muscle can be just as unhealthy as too much fat. This is seen in individuals with chronic diseases like cancer. It can also be present in MONW people. The TEMT plan is designed to prevent, reduce, and reverse sarcopenia.

Beyond the bathroom scale and BMI, there lives a place called Thriving. Thriving happens when you acknowledge your body—skinny, overweight, or in between—recognize the current body you are living in, and choose to honor your body with vigorous daily movement. When you use your muscles daily, your metabolism wakes up; you become physically, mentally, and emotionally stronger; and you help prevent sarcopenia.

We certainly don't want to sound like we're knocking individuals who are naturally thin. Our point is that we all have to work at keeping fit and staying healthy. When we honor our bodies with consistent, daily movement, we set the stage for thriving.

 Dr. James on Sarcopenia
http://www.youtube.com/watch?v=wD37WKEVkfk&list=PLDF2 6DC5254801299

Seeing Our Bodies for What They Are

Compared to fifty years ago, the average American woman has gained about nine inches around her waist and twenty pounds on the scale.

Today, the average American woman is nearly 5′4″ tall, has an average waist size of 37.5 inches, and weighs 166.2 pounds. In the 1960s, the average woman was just over 5′3″ tall, had a waist size of about 24–25 inches and weighed about 120 pounds. The average American man is 5′9″, weighs 195.5 pounds, and has a waist size of 39.7 inches.[2] In 1960, the average man was 5′8.2″ and weighed 168 pounds.[3]

It is time for a reality check.

We want you to love yourself and love your body at every size—but we also want you to live a long, healthy, fulfilled life. This is more difficult to do when you are overweight or obese, or when you depend solely on what you look like to determine your fitness level. We know that over one-third of adults in the United States are obese,[4] and we want to radically downshift that statistic. So get out your calculators, and let's calculate your BMI right now. It's not the best tool out there, neither is it the "be all end all," but it's one way of tracking where you are right in this moment.

• • • • • • • • • • • •

ACTION STEP

Take your height in inches (let's use 70 as an example) and multiply that number by itself (in other words, square it). In our example, that would be: $70 \times 70 = 4900$.

Next, divide your weight in pounds by this number (let's use 175). So, $175 \div 4900 = .035714285$.

Now, multiply this number by 703 to get your BMI. In our example, $703 \times .035714285 = 25.11$. This BMI falls into the overweight category. Here's a BMI guide for you:

Underweight = 18.5 and under
Normal weight = 18.5 to 24.9
Overweight = 25 to 29.9
Obese = 30 or greater

. . . .

Remember, this isn't perfect science, but it is a place to start. If you are extremely fit, BMI is *not* the best tool for measuring fitness (actually, it doesn't measure fitness at all). If your BMI is in the 25 or above range, that doesn't necessarily mean you aren't fit; but you may want to consider other ways of measuring and testing your current fitness and health levels (including a thorough physical with your doctor, body fat percentage measurement, resting metabolic rate, and a stress test). If your BMI falls at 30 or above, it's probably time to make some changes. Love yourself and your body where you are right now, and commit to working toward a healthier lifestyle.

One of the first steps to thriving is loving ourselves right were we are, so focus on health and fitness as an act of loving yourself. Remember, we believe that self-care and self-love are forms of social activism.

Author Check-In

Debra's body image: At 5'2½", I've been challenged with body image for most of my life. For one thing, I have very short legs and my inner thighs have always touched, no matter how much I weigh or how hard I train. I've always had a butt. Some might envy that butt, but not me. My weight actually rarely fluctuates. During times when I have been training for endurance events like marathons or even the Half Ironman Triathlon, I actually gained weight, which was a bit of a frustration for me. It didn't matter that my body-fat percentage had been as low as 15 percent; all I noticed were my inner thighs—actually my thighs in general. It didn't phase me that people complimented the shape of my arms or the flatness of my belly, or asked me if I had been a gymnast (never was). All I knew or cared about was that I had big thighs and my butt was too big. I gained less than twenty-five pounds (this is a good thing) with each pregnancy by eating well and exercising daily, and I lost the pregnancy weight within six weeks of giving birth (also very positive). I have enthusiastically empowered and supported other women in their quest to love themselves, but inside, I struggled with my own acceptance.

There's something about consistently doing the work and taking action that has finally led me to acceptance and self-love. For me, it is in the gift of movement itself, and in the knowing that it is a privilege to have a strong, able body. I am diligent with my workouts; I am strong; I am becoming more flexible; I am happy; and I am so grateful. It comes back to the idea that I am enough. Just like you are enough. It's not about the size of my thighs, the length of my legs, or how much I weigh; it's about the actions I take every day that lead to acceptance and shift my perspective of thriving.

Exercise: Acceptance and Action

You can't change your body just by thinking about it, but you can change the way you think about your body—and you can do something about it if you aren't excited about what you see. What this equates to is acceptance and action.

Acceptance: Accept the things you can't change. Although there are many things you can change about your appearance, you can't change your past or your height (though some would debate this, given that you can wear high heels or lifts; we're talking about your actual height). If going on an ice cream binge got your thighs where they are today, or a broken leg kept you out of the gym and you got a little softer around the middle—well, that was then and this is now. There is nothing you can do to fix or change those facts. What you *can* do is accept the experience(s) as a learning tool for moving forward, and take action now.

Action: Action may look a lot like work, but exercise is another non-negotiable reality when it comes to Thriving. If you are having trouble getting started or getting motivated to exercise, think of the rush of endorphins (feel-good chemicals) that you will enjoy post-workout. Think of your powerful *why*—your intrinsic motivation for exercising. Get to bed at a decent hour and have a plan for exercising tomorrow!

When we lovingly and willingly accept our bodies, and are willing to take action to shift what no longer serves us, we set ourselves up for positive action and Thriving.

10

MOVE Your Mindset

There are a thousand-plus excuses for why you may not be exercising—you don't have the time; you can't find an exercise you enjoy; you're too old to start running; you can't do yoga because you're not flexible enough, and the classes you would take are never at the right time; and so on. But you are a resourceful person! No matter how legitimate the reasons may feel when you say them, you can find a reasonable solution. Exercise just needs to be a priority. And once you bring the intention to exercise to your daily life, you will find both the time and the way around the reasons you've previously used to avoid it.

Move and Be Moved

Exercise is key, not just for the heart but also for the head. Exercise shifts our physical well-being as well as our emotional well-being. People who don't exercise often isolate themselves from others, or become insecure due to their perceived lack of coordination or athleticism. Once you start exercising and seeing changes in your body and mind, self-confidence starts to increase. You begin to think more clearly and start setting other lifestyle goals due to the energy you get from exercising. Exercise provides opportunities to network, make new friends, socialize—connect with people. On the other hand, if you need some quiet downtime, activities like swimming, biking, running, and yoga provide an awesome space for reflection and "me time."

Rates of depression are at an all-time high in this country. Anxiety is also on the rise. But something as simple as walking for twenty to thirty minutes a day may keep depression at bay.

One of the coolest things about exercise is how it affects the brain. On one hand, exercise supports the creation of new brain cells, which is stimulating, but at the same time, it can induce a state of calm.[1] Exercise helps relieve and reduce stress by reducing cortisol and adrenaline in the body. And it elevates mood and reduces pain through the production of endorphins.

Studies have shown that regular exercise can ease some cancer-related side effects, including fatigue, depression, anxiety, pain, and sleeping troubles.[2] Exercise may also reduce the fatality rate among women diagnosed with breast cancer. This is true for women diagnosed with stage I, II, or III breast cancer. One particular study, published in the *Journal of the American Medical Association* (JAMA), showed that breast cancer patients who began to walk thirty to sixty minutes per day were 50 percent less likely to die from the disease than their sedentary counterparts. The greatest benefit occurred in women who walked an average of three to five hours per week at an average pace.[3]

Embrace Sweat

While any movement is fabulous (and we love incidental fitness), you should dive in and learn to embrace some strenuous exercise that makes you sweat.

Sweating is usually a result of an increased heart rate and body temperature. This accelerates metabolism and increases circulation; and increased circulation helps to move toxins out through the pores. This not only helps the look and feel of the skin but sweating may also give a boost to the immune system. As the body heats up, white blood cells are generated, strengthening the immune system.

In short, sweating just makes us feel better. The increase in body temperature helps the body to relax as it dispels stress throughout.

Dress the Part

There is something about looking the part and feeling good about ourselves that can get us through potentially challenging times. We are reminded of the expression "fake it till you make it." Another way of saying this is "acting *as if*," like we did in THINK earlier. No matter what you want to call it, it is all about generating confidence when and where you might not be feeling so confident normally. What you wear during exercise may make a difference in how you feel before, during, and after your workout. Exercise clothes need to fit well, wick moisture, be comfortable—and it doesn't hurt if they help you feel good lookin' too!

Researchers at Northwestern University introduced a term called *enclothed cognition*, which describes the idea that what we wear influences our psychology.[4] Enclothed cognition explains two phenomena that occur when we dress the part: (1) the symbolic meaning of the clothes and (2) the physical experience of wearing them.

What you wear can affect how you perceive yourself and how others perceive you. Think of professional athletes and sports teams. The Oakland Raiders, for example, wear black uniforms that contribute to their intimidating reputation around the NFL. Many athletes who don't have a set uniform already wear what they consider to be their "power color" while playing. For example, Tiger Woods usually wears red on the last day of a tournament because his mom said it was his power color.

The clothing we wear can also affect our performance. For example, it is important to wear clothing that will wick away moisture when you exercise. Wicking fabrics take moisture away from the skin and to the outside of the fabric. This helps your body regulate its temperature so it can perform at a higher level. Cotton can be comfortable, but it doesn't wick moisture from the body. In fact, if you sweat a lot in a cotton shirt (we've all been there), chances of chafing and being generally uncomfortable skyrocket. Types of wicking fabric may contain polypropylene, silk, wool, a synthetic blend, or you'll see trademarked wicking fabrics, like Coolmax and Supplex.

Layering is another key thing to keep in mind when exercising. You need to dress for the climate of your workout, taking into account whether you are exercising inside or outside. As long as your bottom layer is comprised of a fabric that wicks, you should be good to go.

Wearing clothing that fits well is also important. Though it's totally understandable to be self-conscious, especially when first starting out, excess fabric tends to increase the risk of chafing, and it restricts movement with its bulkiness.

Author Check-In

Debra's shoes: I have a lot of experience in exercise-appropriate gear. When I decided to get into tennis in my thirties, I signed up for what I thought was a recreation-center class. Turns out I had joined a league and ranked myself slightly above where I belonged in that setting. I wore my running shoes, shorts, and a t-shirt to my first practice and nearly got heckled by the coach. I actually thought she and my teammates were joking when they said I couldn't wear "those" shoes—but they weren't. Sure enough, I went out right away and bought actual "tennis" shoes, and eventually, slowly but surely, dressed the part with the tennis skirts and tanks. I do believe it made a difference in my game, which has come a long way since then.

When I started swimming and training for my first triathlon I didn't have any of the proper attire that "real" triathletes had; I didn't even own a swim cap. Dressing the part not only gave me more confidence to continue with the sport but it improved my performance as well. I may have felt uncomfortable the first time I put on a wetsuit, but it helped me become more confident, giving me the courage to train in open waters.

• • • • • • • • • • • •

ACTION STEP

We're neither expecting nor suggesting that you go out and drop a small fortune on exercise clothing. Instead, check out your closet for shirts made from wicking fabrics (synthetic or blended fiber), both short-sleeved and long; and check out old pajamas, sweats, and other clothes you may have kept around for yard work or the like. You can also:

- Compare prices online—you'll find a lot of bargains this way. The downside is that you can't try on the clothes before you buy them, and fit is super important. You may want to check out shipping costs for returns before purchasing.
- Shop clearance racks at sporting goods stores. You can often find exercise clothing for all sports at a generous discount. End of season is also a good time to look for deals. Thrift shops are another option.
- Don't get caught up in name brands. Choose lesser-known brands that offer the same functionality at better prices.
- Join email lists, and sign up for customer loyalty programs that offer points or rewards for purchases made at the store. You will often find that discount coupons arrive via email, and you can use them to shop online or in store.

There is something to be said for dressing the part and stepping into the role of your desires. When it comes down to it, wear things that make you feel good *and* are suited to what you are doing.

. . . .

Efficiency Counts

One of the most common excuses for not exercising is lack of time. This is a major misconception. When you engage in high-intensity interval training (HIIT), you can have an effective workout in ten minutes. The other thing you can do is break up your workout into several smaller workouts throughout the day.

Do not give in to the idea that exercise only works when you have an extra hour to spare. This is a limited belief that doesn't serve you. Make exercise a priority and schedule it into your day. Get creative. If it works for you to wake up a bit earlier, go for it—you're more likely to stick with exercise when you do it first thing. If getting in ten to fifteen minutes on your lunch break works, go for it. Exercise works whenever you make it happen. So get creative, and go for it!

. . . .

ACTION STEP

Perform ten minutes of HIIT immediately after you wake up. This may look like jump roping intervals, driveway sprints, mountain climbers alternating with burpees, or jumping jacks interspersed with push-ups. Follow with a healthy snack or protein-enhanced shake. At lunchtime, or some other time during the day, get out for a fifteen-minute walk (with coworkers, your dog, your kids—whatever works). Before dinner, do ten minutes of stretching or yoga to unwind. The next day, wake up and do five minutes of warm-up calisthenics followed by ten minutes of weight lifting, or ten minutes of resistance training that uses your body weight (push-ups, sit-ups, pull-ups, tricep dips). Before or after dinner, put on a few of your favorite dance tunes and shake your booty.

You need to schedule the time. Set a reminder on your cell phone if it helps; or ask family members or friends to join you. Any time you can squeeze in five, ten, fifteen minutes of movement, do it. The efforts will accumulate, and your mind and body will reap the benefits.

. . . .

Remember, *any* time is the right time when it comes to exercise. In our house, we are morning people, and exercising first thing in the morning really works well for us; it sets us up for success throughout the day. We understand that not everyone is a morning person, but the earlier you get it in, the greater the likelihood that you will get it done. Despite great intentions to exercise "later," life often gets in the way, and exercise falls to the wayside. So, schedule it in. Make exercise a non-negotiable task on your daily to-do list.

 Best Time to Exercise
http://www.youtube.com/watch?v=0todyZHz4jU&list=PLDF2
6DC5254801299

Incidental Fitness

There are many powerful and positive ways to begin incorporating fitness into your life. You can begin by simply using your body. Push-ups, squats, lunges, pull-ups, and other exercises require no special equipment or gym. We love creating opportunities for incidental fitness throughout the day. If you are waiting for your morning cup of tea to steep or your coffee to brew, why not drop to the ground and do five to ten push-ups;

or push up from the countertop in your kitchen if you are new to push-ups. While you are brushing your teeth, perform a series of modified squats. Look for chances throughout the day to get moving!

Author Check-In

Debra's incidental fitness: Our favorite moments of incidental fitness definitely happen with our dogs. James and I are committed to getting them out for walks every day and go together as often as we can. On the weekends, we take them for longer hikes. We're also avid skiers and bikers (we call this incidental fitness since we do these things out of enjoyment rather than obligation). In the summer, we love to work in the yard and play a little frisbee after dinner; and in the winter, we get in our fair share of snow shoveling.

Blue Zones

We are big fans and students of the research of people who are living in the Blue Zones, as identified by Dan Buettner and published in his book of the same title.[5] Blue Zones are communities where common elements of lifestyle, diet, and outlook have led to an amazing length and quality of life. These communities have been studied by researchers at the National Institute on Aging and researchers all over the world. People living in Blue Zones tend to engage in daily, low-intensity exercise that may just look a lot like activities of daily living (gardening, snow shoveling, walking or biking to work, housecleaning, and so on).

Okinawans live in a Blue Zone, for example. They spend hours in the garden, where they exhibit key attributes of exercise and stress reduction, including bending, reaching, and pulling; weeding a patch of soil; seeding a new bed; or harvesting fresh and beautiful fruits and veggies. Hours in the garden may not raise your heart rate like a series of wind sprints, but they will have a powerful effect on stimulating key health-inducing hormones. Gardening will also decrease the levels of hormones that challenge your longevity and overall well-being.

Too many of us are spending a lot of time in traffic when a walk would do us good. We may drive around looking for the closest parking spot when the one farther away would nourish both our body and our mind. The beauty and blessing of moving naturally is that it can—and will—become a powerful and seamless part of daily living once you set the intention to do it.

Moving naturally can easily be a part of your daily routine. Perhaps it looks like taking a walk with your morning tea or coffee. Perhaps it's the small or large garden that you tend daily with love and zeal. Insist upon getting outdoors and discipline yourself to do so after dinner—to allow for connection with a loved one or just sweet downtime for yourself. Buddhists have a walking meditation practice, which is simply walking mindfully in silence.

What moving naturally may lack in intensity is made up in serenity. Gandhi said, "There is more to life than increasing its speed." Allow for the lessons of Blue Zone communities and peoples to teach you the law of doing well with less. Get outside of the "gym rat" mentality and courageously choose to play in the natural world with passion and a grateful heart.

When you want to add more structure to your movement program, you may purchase some dumbbells, or get creative with soup cans. We like to improvise with household items for things like bicep curls, tricep kickbacks, chest presses, or shoulder presses. Water bottles also work well as impromptu dumbbells.

• • • • • • • • • • • • •

ACTION STEP

Next time you find yourself standing or sitting, consider the ways in which you could be more active:

- Do squats when watching the morning traffic report.
- Drop down and perform five push-ups every time you get off the couch to go to the kitchen.
- Bicep dips using the counter when making tea or waiting for coffee to brew.
- Put on music when you're doing the dishes, getting ready for an evening out, or cleaning the house, to encourage you to move faster and expend energy.
- Buy or borrow a balance ball (a.k.a. exercise ball) and sit on it when you are working from home or watching TV.
- Plant a small garden or join a community garden.
- Choose a new part of town or trail to explore by foot or bike.
- Volunteer for a trail cleanup or food drive.

Exercise: Get Moving

Still holding on to excuses for not exercising? We believe you are more than capable (and deserving) of thriving, not just surviving. Here are some ideas to help you get moving:

- Write down at least five activities (on small pieces of paper) that you are willing to commit to at least trying. You may include walking, running, dancing, biking, swimming, weight lifting, yoga, Crossfit, or even doing a home-based DVD exercise program. Now, place those papers in a small bowl or a hat, and place it somewhere that you will see it every morning.

- Next, find at least two sets of clothing, two pairs of socks, and a pair of decent sneakers (cross-training or running shoes) that you can wear for exercise. Set them out where you will see them.
- Get to bed thirty minutes earlier than you are used to and set the alarm for thirty minutes earlier than you are used to waking up.
- Once your alarm goes off, reach into the bowl (or hat) and pick out one piece of paper. That is what you'll be doing today. Put on one of the outfits you set out, and lace up your shoes; it's time to get moving. Give yourself at least fifteen minutes of exercise; and if the moment moves you to continue—and you have the extra time—go for it.

11

MOVE Your Routine

There are infinite possibilities when it comes to movement and exercise. And just like diets and eating plans, some ways of moving are more beneficial than others. When it comes down to it, consider the whole package of TEMT: you want to Think about eating and exercising mindfully, and always be present to your intentions when it comes to your health; you want to Eat in line with your eating personality but also in a healthful way that cuts the risk for diseases of lifestyle, and ups your Thriving factor; and you want to Move in ways that complement your intentions and your eating.

Author Check-In

James's moving experience: Upon meeting my wife over twenty years ago, she inspired me to add a new twist to my workouts by taking my love of exercise outside of the gym on Friday nights. The place was a dance studio called Body Moves, where they taught Nia (a nonimpact, sensory-based movement practice), yoga, and something called the "5Rhythms / Sweat Your Prayers."

The 5Rhythms practice is a movement-meditation practice created in the 1970s by the late Gabrielle Roth.

Just to set the stage, I am not a "dancer." I love to dance, but I do not have any sense of timing or rhythm. On my first Friday night at Body Moves, however, I walked into a sea of beautiful, barefoot people fully going for it—whirling and twirling with unbridled spirit and freedom. I was instantly reminded of being at a Grateful Dead concert (without the extracurricular substances).

The class was based on Roth's life work, and this was a revelation to me. I learned about the opportunity that movement gives to express, to release, and to become more open and connected to the deepest parts of my being, and I was hooked.

We've been building a foundation for thriving from the beginning of this book, and now it's time to look at some of the more effective ways we can Move—and how you can start to incorporate those into your life. Let's start with a few basics about our favorite, most-effective workout strategies.

High-Intensity Interval Training (HIIT)

A number of physiological processes take place when we exercise, one of which is the secretion of growth hormone (GH). GH is produced in the pituitary gland, stimulating growth, and cellular regeneration and reproduction. GH is what helps us grow during childhood, and it is probably most widely known as a hormone that increases lean muscle mass and reduces body fat. Decreased GH levels in the body have been linked to decreased muscle mass and tone, weight gain, decreased sex drive, decreased bone density, increased formation of wrinkles, decreased skin elasticity, and decreased energy.[1]

GH is usually more abundant in the body during our teens and early twenties, and tends to wane as we get older. GH levels can also decrease when we are sedentary. A highly refined diet, rich in sugar and processed foods, will suppress the release of GH into the bloodstream. As an injectable, prescriptive therapy, GH has been touted as the ultimate antiaging solution and panacea for all things related to beauty. Approved by the US Food and Drug Administration (FDA), physicians are allowed to prescribe GH to treat many health conditions, including multiple sclerosis, colitis, and fibromyalgia.[2] Unfortunately, there aren't a lot of clinical trials to substantiate its use outside of GH deficiency, so we suggest optimizing GH levels naturally.

The best and most efficient way to increase GH naturally—and get it to release at the highest levels—is high-intensity interval training (HIIT). HIIT, sometimes referred to as sprint training, is an intense cardiovascular exercise because it powerfully works the heart and lungs. Some well-known training methods that incorporate HIIT: Tabata training, Fartlek, and CrossFit.

The Tabata Interval Workout

The Tabata interval workout was based on an experiment by Professor Izumi Tabata and colleagues in 1996. Originally performed with speed skaters, Tabata's method has gained tremendous following in fitness circles for its supreme fat-burning power and ease of implementation. A Tabata workout involves choosing an exercise (bike, treadmill, jumping rope, squats, jumping lunges, jumping jacks, mountain climbers, box jumps) and performing the exercise at the highest intensity you can manage for twenty seconds; then resting for ten seconds; then repeating eight to twenty times. This is an extremely efficient and effective workout.

Muscle Confusion

Perhaps you are already exercising most days (if so, good for you!). If you've been doing this for half your life, though, it may be time to switch things up.

When we do the same thing every day, the body adjusts, muscles adapt, and over time, the exercise can become ineffective in terms of seeing any change in body composition, energy levels, or improved fitness levels. Fortunately, in the world of athletics, there is already a solution—a concept known as *muscle confusion*. Muscle confusion is one of the best ways to crash through a fitness plateau. And it is all about varying exercises, repetitions, and weights.

So for all of you athletes, chances are you can take it up a notch. Whether that looks like taking a new class, training for an endurance event, increasing the number of repetitions, or increasing the amount of weight, mixing it up will re-energize your body and mind, and keep you motivated over the long term.

HIIT workouts are very efficient, averaging from five to thirty minutes per session. One way to think about or engage in HIIT is with sprinting (this can be done by running, biking, or swimming). You sprint for thirty to forty-five seconds, then cool down by walking (or slowing your pace) for twenty seconds. Repeat this process for ten or twenty minutes, depending on how much time you have. Then follow up the sprinting with resistance exercise, using free weights, machines, or your body weight.

Author Check-In

James's first HIIT: When I was growing up and playing sports, if we lost or performed poorly, our coaches used to "wake us up" (or help us to remember to "play smarter and harder") by making us do wind sprints, or "suicides." I used to dread them and did my best to run them as fast as possible—to get them over with. Funny thing, in looking back, I remember always feeling "high" after they were done, possibly because of the fact that they were over with. Or maybe it was because they also made for a mindful mix of chemicals that we now know makes us happier, smarter, and perhaps even younger?

We love HIIT because of its efficiency. And the more we research vitality and aging, the more it seems like HIIT is the only way to go.

This has been a huge wake-up call for us. For more than half of our adult lives, both of us have participated in a wide range of endurance events. From half-marathons and marathons to the half Ironman and full Ironman triathlons, we've set our goals high and nearly burned out achieving them. As much as we enjoy the personal satisfaction we get from competing in and completing endurance events, we have found that we can still achieve a high level of fitness through working out efficiently and HIIT training. We feel better, look better, and still enjoy participating in sprint events and charity runs several times a year—all without really having to put in a lot of training because our base fitness is maintained with HIIT.

Fast-forward a few years, to the future us, and we are still participating in fun fitness events (like 5K or 10K fun runs or sprint-distance triathlons), but we don't log the same number of hours training as we did in the past. Now, we combine HIIT with yoga and other fun exercises, like tennis, Zumba, mountain biking, skiing, and Nia, and get so much more out of our workouts. We feel more energized, our immune systems stay strong, and we have a lot more time for family and friends.

While HIIT is shown to stimulate release of GH, recent research indicates that endurance training actually results in *decreased* GH levels.[3] Resistance training with weights also increases secretion of GH, which is why we like to combine HIIT with some weight training. Though the response is stronger in your twenties and thirties, the good news is that you can still stimulate release of GH well into your seventies. So for greater workout efficiency, give HIIT a try.

Getting rid of fat and building muscle isn't supposed to be easy; you need to want it, and you need to work for it. If all of this is new to you, we definitely recommend first talking to your doctor and also engaging a certified fitness professional who can take you through some different HIIT routines. We are somewhat biased toward CrossFit (we love it), as CrossFit is suitable for beginners and super athletes alike. We also think it's a great way to bring a community feel to your workout. Even better, CrossFit gyms are sprouting up all across the country, so you may find one right in your neck of the woods.

 Dr. James Demonstrates Sprinting
http://www.youtube.com/watch?v=ShTx-nWrpWQ&list=PLD
F26DC5254801299

Embrace Resistance with Strength

Lean muscle mass (basically muscle without the fat) is an independent factor for healthy aging. One of the most important secrets to Thriving and aging gracefully is building and maintaining muscle. Muscle burns calories exponentially more efficiently than fat. It keeps us strong, active, and balanced. Muscle helps us appear and feel more youthful, gives us confidence, protects and strengthens our bones. Strength training uses weight resistance—in the form of dumbbells, machines, kettlebells, or body weight—to increase lean muscle mass. And it can result in muscle hypertrophy, which means an increase in size. This is the purpose behind bodybuilding, but strength training isn't just for bodybuilders.

Testosterone in Women

We understand that women in particular may have concerns about getting big or bulky from strength training—but that's not what strength training will do for you. Testosterone is responsible for the large increase of muscle mass that you can see with competitive male bodybuilders. Women's testosterone levels are a fraction of men's. If you are picturing female bodybuilders who look overly muscular or even manly, there is a likelihood that she is using some kind of exogenous hormone therapy to develop those muscles. "Natural" female bodybuilders have incredibly beautiful physiques with long lean muscles, not bulky.

Author Check-In

Debra's strength training: I can't tell you how many times I've heard women use the excuse of not lifting weights because they don't want to look like a "gross bodybuilder." Becoming "over muscled" takes an amazing level of lifting, and possibly involves using steroids and other anabolic agents. The likelihood of ever becoming that big from doing normal lifting and resistance training is next to impossible. James has been lifting weights since he was a teenager. Jack LaLanne inspired him by suggesting that that with every push-up, bicep curl, and squat, we can imagine that we are lifting the weight of the world off of our minds and shoulders. I have also been strength training with weights since my teens, and never once has anyone accused me of looking too masculine. The metaphors and the real empowerment that come from weight lifting and resistance training are remarkable for mind, body, and overall aging and longevity.

• • • •

Part III: MOVE

Many folks here in the United States have chosen comfort over longevity. Although there can be other explanations for sarcopenia, aging and inactivity are the two biggies. During our thirties, most adults start to lose muscle, which is why strength training becomes essential. Loss of muscle means loss of strength; and that means loss of protection for bones, loss of stamina, and more.

Strength training will help reduce body fat; strengthen bones; and reduce the risk of chronic diseases like heart disease, type 2 diabetes, obesity, and arthritis. It is an essential component of overall fitness and optimum wellness.

The basic principle of strength training involves lifting weights or using body weight to achieve an increase in strength and endurance. This is achieved via a number of repetitions (reps), which are cycles of lifting and lowering weights (or doing push-ups or pull-ups for example). We usually recommend six to twelve repetitions per cycle.

The completion of one cycle of repetitions is referred to as a set. Usually two to five sets of repetitions are performed one after another, with no more than a thirty-second break in between sets, for the most effective workout. We like sets of six to twelve repetitions because that number appears to be key for developing muscle strength, size, and endurance. And just to clarify, when we talk about lifting weights, the weights should feel heavy; strength training isn't supposed to be easy. It will challenge you physically and mentally. But we Thrive on all levels—mental, physical, emotional, spiritual—when we are challenged and when we work hard.

Lifting weights can be a game changer for those aged sixty and beyond. Resistance work and weight training improve balance and flexibility, which can prevent falls and broken bones. And it can improve the mind. A meta-analysis of forty-nine studies investigating the role of resistance exercise on lean muscle mass in adults aged fifty and beyond concluded that resistance exercise is effective for improving lean muscle mass in this population.[4] Boston University studied a group of older adults (average age of sixty-eight years) over a twelve-week program of strength training three times per week. This group was measured for a variety of fitness, psychological, and cognitive functions. Muscle strength improved by nearly 40 percent; body fat decreased by 3 percent; and the participants experienced improvements in mood, fitness, and anxiety.[5]

You will see vastly improved results when you combine interval/speed work with strength and resistance training. The key to getting great results is to move and move quickly. The downtime in between sets should be less than a minute and, if possible, inside of thirty seconds. The days of being in the gym, logging sets and miles for hours, are over. Move fast, sweat a lot, and know that when you are done, you will feel rejuvenated, empowered, and exhausted—all at the same time. Treat this as an opportunity to play.

Author Check-In

Debra's "bat wing" solution: One of the most common questions I get from women is, "How do I get rid of my bat wings?" Of course, they are referring to that extra skin and fat that hangs down below your tricep, on the underside of your arm. It's what jiggles when you're waving hello or good-bye to someone. It may also be referred to as saggy or floppy tricep syndrome. The most effective exercises you can do to prevent the bat-wing phenomenon are push-ups, tricep dips, tricep kickbacks, and tricep extensions.

 Dr. Debra On Triceps Exercises
http://youtu.be/Ddh4SGEPcOA

• • • • • • • • • • • •

ACTION STEP

Try to incorporate strength training at least four times per week. Here are some ways to do that:

- Combine dumbbell squats with jumping rope. Do 10 to 15 reps of squats, with or without dumbbells, and follow with 30 seconds of rope jumping. Repeat 3 to 5 sets.
- Combine dumbbell press, barbell press, or push-ups with speed punching. Do 10 to 15 reps of press/push-ups with 30 seconds of speed/shadow punching. Repeat for 3 to 5 sets.
- Combine pull-ups with jumping jacks. Do as many pull-ups as possible and follow with 30 seconds of fast-paced jumping jacks. Repeat for 3 to 5 sets.
- Combine bicep curls with weights or bands with mountain climbers. Do 10 to 15 reps of bicep curls with 30 seconds of mountain climbers. Repeat for 3 to 5 sets.

You can do these exercises in the above order the first week and then do them from bottom to top the second week; and the third, mix it up again. You can make this workout as easy or as hard as you wish. It is not about destroying yourself; it is about taking yourself to the edge and doing it well. Do not sacrifice form for speed. You will see a noticeable improvement with your strength and endurance in as little as a few weeks. Your body will be leaner, and your confidence and trust in your body will soar.

• • • • • • • • • • • •

 Dr. James on Strength Training and Cognitive Function
http://www.youtube.com/watch?v=l94iAViB-
L2I&list=PLDF26DC5254801299

Yoga, Nia, and Zumba

Running can be great for your cardiovascular health, but make sure your hips and knees can take it by focusing on form and not distance. If running isn't your thing, there are many fun and invigorating ways to work up a sweat. Yoga, Nia, and Zumba are movement practices led by experienced and certified trainers (hopefully), usually in a group setting within a fitness studio. Each one builds strength and stamina, and is the perfect complement to any fitness regimen.

Yoga has an incredibly rich history that dates back to around 500 BCE, though its exact origin is up for debate. It is thought to have originated in India, and it continues to play a prominent role in the philosophical cultures of Hinduism and Buddhism. Our favorite interpretation of the word yoga itself means "union." The process and practice of yoga is a union of inner consciousness with Universal consciousness.

Yoga came to the United States in the late nineteenth century but didn't gain popularity until the mid-1980s. Some people still mistake yoga for a religious practice, but yoga can be as spiritual a practice as you want to make of it, just as running or swimming can. There is no particular religious creed that you must ascribe to in order to participate; there is no political agenda in yoga. Your yoga practice can be highly physical, restorative, meditative, or all of the above. That's just part of why we love it.

In yoga, we move through a series of postures (*asanas*) that not only support balance, alignment, heat, and flexibility in the body but also peace of mind. Yoga supports every aspect of optimum wellness, lowering the risk of heart disease, helping to control symptoms of type 2 diabetes, decreasing the severity of menopausal symptoms, reducing chronic back pain, relieving stress, managing depression and anxiety, and improving sleep quality. It has also been shown to positively effect all phases of the menstrual cycle and may be an effective management for premenstrual stress or tension.[6]

We encourage you to give yoga your consideration and try to incorporate it into your everyday fitness plan. This could be for five minutes or ninety minutes. You may discover that you prefer doing yoga in a heated studio, in the privacy of your home, or right in your work cubicle; there are several online resources available to support your practice. Many are free or charge a small monthly fee, which basically pays for itself after you've done one class. We really like yogaglo.com because there is a wide variety of styles, duration, teachers, and levels to choose from. All you need is a computer or tablet and, preferably, a yoga mat and block. Your local library may also have yoga DVDs available.

Yoga and stretching are good for muscles after a workout, and they can get your mind in the perfect place for meditation, prayer, and visualizing. When you're all amped up after a busy day or an evening meeting, yoga is a great way to help you wind down.

Pranayama

If you've ever gone to a vinyasa class—the most common type of yoga class in the United States currently—*ujjayi* (victorious breath) was most likely used, to help connect your breath to your movement (another aspect of union used in most yoga practices).

Other common *pranayama* include *kapalabhati* (literally "skull shining" breath), *nadi shodhana* (alternate nostril breathing), and *sama vritti* (equal-parts breath). Patañjali, the sage who collected the yoga sutras, wrote that building on your yoga practice by beginning a pranayama practice is a big step, requiring a lot of strength and concentration. This is what we say: if you're just starting out with pranayama, stick with the simple equal-parts breath, as some pranayama isn't recommended for people with certain health issues; and it can be an advanced practice that affects your organs.

A simple five or ten minutes of yoga breathing (*pranayama*) and gentle stretching can ease you back into hormonal harmony, and put your mind and body in sleep-receiving mode. Pranayama consists of a slow, deep inhale, suspending of the breath, and then a slow exhale. There are a variety of ways to practice pranayama, and various yoga schools and traditions practice pranayama differently.

• • • • • • • • • • • •

ACTION STEP

Practice pranayama by sitting quietly for five minutes and focusing on your breath.

- Inhale slowly through the nose, with your mouth closed, while counting to five.
- Exhale through the nose, counting to five at the same pace.
- After you feel comfortable, and the breath feels smooth while doing this, add in holding your breath at the top of the breath (after a full inhale) for the same count.
- Continue so you are practicing this pranayama for a total of ten minutes.

You don't want to hold the breath at your exhale, as that is an advanced practice that can create disharmony in the body if you aren't trained in what to do. But holding it at the top of the breath (after a full inhale) helps you stay in the moment.

As you do this, consider that part of the breath at which your body feels most comfortable, and stay aware of your body and mental state as you do this practice. This breath is called *sama vritti*, or equal-parts breath. It calms the nervous system, increases focus, reduces stress, and helps your body achieve balance.

• • • • • • • • • • • •

Yoga may be your primary form of exercise or it may serve as an awesome cross-training, stretching, or relaxation practice to augment your existing fitness routine. There are an endless variety of asana series and yoga schools to choose from. We recommend you try several types and teachers to find a practice that is right for you. We've known too many folks who tried one class and decided yoga wasn't for them. It may take a while to find the right practice to suit your personality and style. But once you do, we believe you'll be incredibly happy to have stuck with it.

At the end of most yoga practices, we end in a pose called *savasana*, also known as corpse pose. Savasana anchors the practice and is like a reward for a job well done. It is also a great posture to set the tone for deep sleep. To practice savasana, lie flat on your back on the floor (not on your bed). Allow your legs to be about twelve to eighteen inches apart and your feet to fall naturally to the side. Arms are alongside the body, palms facing up. Roll shoulders back and under. From here, practice releasing any tension you may be feeling with each exhalation. Keep your belly soft. This is a mysteriously simple and powerful pose, and can help calm the body and mind any time of day.

Nia is the next powerful practice we'd like to discuss. Nia was developed by Debbie Rosas and Carlos AyaRosas in 1983. It began as a barefoot, nonimpact, aerobics-style dance class and has naturally evolved into a purposeful, body-centered awareness movement that draws from elements of dance, yoga, martial arts, and other healing art forms. Nia choreography is based on fifty-two core movements and is appropriate for every shape and size, all levels of athletic ability, and all ages. An average Nia class lasts about an hour and is facilitated by a Nia-certified trainer. (Nia teacher trainings are offered as "intensives," which consist of progressive belt levels, beginning with White Belt training and followed by Green, Blue, Brown, and Black.)

Author Check-In

Debra's love of Nia: I will admit I am partial to Nia. The Nia headquarters are based in Portland, OR, and I discovered Nia while

James and I were in our last year of naturopathic medical school there. I attended Debbie Rosas's classes whenever I could. Nia was not only invigorating for my body but it was also healing for my spirit. At the time, I was working, delivering babies, and going to school, but I had also lost my dad unexpectedly. It was all I could do to get up everyday, let alone function. My dad and I were very close, and his passing was devastating. But Nia kept me going; kept me sane, whole, and centered. As a graduation gift to myself, I completed the White Belt teacher training. A few years later in Colorado, I completed my Blue Belt and enjoyed teaching Nia for several years. Nia fulfills part of my passion and purpose, and I will always be grateful for its gifts.

To add a little spice, we bring you Zumba. Zumba fitness came to the US market in 2001. Each Zumba class is like a dance party—fast-paced, choreographed, and exhilarating. While, understandably, some people are intimidated by this, even the most uncoordinated of individuals can enjoy Zumba and should give it a try if given the opportunity. Like Nia, Zumba fuses many dance styles, and the brand has expanded to include everything from Aquatic Zumba to chair-based Zumba, Zumba Kids, and more. Zumba also offers DVD workouts, and chances are that your local library may have a copy you can try.

Your Moving Personality

Defining your fitness personality may be even more important than defining your eating personality. We think of your fitness personality as describing how you typically operate in your life, and we think of your exercise personality as defining specific regimens that work for you. For James, he is highly motivated and feels at home in a gym with plenty of free weights, medicine balls, pull-up bars, and so on. He is a physical-fitness disciple. But exercise can truly be any sort of enjoyable physical activity (best when it increases your heart rate). The key to staying fit is to find out what you enjoy and what motivates you. We'll outline a few fitness personalities here:

- **The Disciple:** This physical-fitness enthusiast (like James) will likely enjoy HIIT, going to the gym, running, biking, lifting weights, swimming, and participating in any other challenging physical endeavors.

- **The Spiritual Warrior:** If you are drawn more to the body–mind component of exercise, you may enjoy yoga, tai chi, walking, Pilates, martial arts, or Nia, all of which are sensory-based movement practices. Workouts provide introspection for you. This fitness personality may also enjoy long-distance running and swimming.

- **The Chameleon:** You may prefer the camaraderie or pace of a fitness class. There are so many different types of classes to choose from, and you can find most of them online or at the nearest recreation or fitness center. Jazzercise, Zumba, spinning, boot camp, kickboxing, and circuit training are all examples of this. Having a variety to choose from is great for people who like to change things up on a regular basis. We've had friends take up ballet in their sixties. Why not?

- **The Team Player:** Perhaps you played sports when you were younger and want to get back into it. There are plenty of adult leagues for soccer, tennis, lacrosse, hockey, basketball, volleyball—again, the local recreation center is one of the best places to find out what is going on locally. And if there is a sport you've always wanted to play, it's never too late to start. Tennis is a wonderful sport to take up at any age—you can be part of a tennis league well into your eighties.

- **The Zen Mover:** You are a person who likes to plug into the same routine every day, like working out at the same time every day. Maybe you love to listen to music while you work out, or you love to read but don't have much time to yourself. You might enjoy working out on a treadmill, elliptical trainer, or stationary bike (this is where Debra finds time to read magazines, for example). You can also adjust your level of effort and work in intervals to make a more effective workout.

- **The Tree Hugger:** There is another very important type of fitness that some may think doesn't qualify as exercise. We might agree that moving naturally wouldn't prepare you to run a marathon, but it may set you up for a long, vital life. In fact, moving naturally is what happens when you maintain an active lifestyle—naturally. In communities where people live the longest and are the happiest, moving naturally is a common denominator. Walking the dog, gardening, cleaning house, hiking, golfing, shoveling snow—these are all forms of functional fitness. They happen as a result of your natural lifestyle, and they certainly count for something!

- **The Adventure Lover:** And for those of you who love spontaneity, crave the outdoors and adventure, there's cross-country skiing, snowshoeing, hiking, mountain biking, rock climbing, surfing, roller-skating or Rollerblading, kayaking, and stand-up paddling.

Your options are limitless. Maybe the list above will give you fresh ideas and inspire you to try something new. Maybe you've been a routine exerciser your entire adult life and are ready to move into the adventurer mode. Maybe you had given up on moving regularly simply because you aren't a gym goer or a class lover, but now you see all the other options. Whatever the case, figure out what really suits you and how you can go about implementing that knowledge in your daily life. Exercise is readily available for us at all times. It is a privilege to move your body; ask anyone whose movement has been compromised. Don't forsake the gift.

Author Check-In

Debra's exercise routine: I've got to say that I'm usually up for any and all of these exercises. I'm disciplined but not obsessed; I'm adventurous but not a thrill seeker. I sometimes love the camaraderie of a team or a class format and just as often find that I want more of an introspective workout. I think that, for women, this is pretty normal. I like to move along with the cycles of my body and listen to what I need in any given moment. Usually it's a good sweat, but on occasion, I will honor myself with a simple walk, restorative yoga, or tennis with friends.

Exercise: You've Got a Friend

We've introduced you to many forms of exercise and hopefully you've learned something new. Here's what we would like you to consider:

Call up a friend or family member (that you actually enjoy spending time with) and make a date for HIIT. Agree to meet at a park, a set of stairs, a gym, your driveway, or a trail, and decide ahead of time how long you will train and what it will consist of. We would suggest a goal of fifteen minutes HIIT to get started. You can either take turns doing intervals or you can do them together, making it more of a competition. You should definitely break a sweat and experience an elevated heart rate. Just take care of yourself; and if you are someone with known asthma or exercise-induced asthma, make sure to bring along your inhaler. Also bring plenty of water, and dress in layers. Chances are you'll heat up quickly, but you may appreciate an extra layer when you're cooling down.

After your HIIT session, support each other with strength challenges. Have a contest for who can hold plank the longest (plank is your position at the top of a push-up), or see who can do the most push-ups. Wrap up your time together with at least five minutes of stretching. If you are already familiar and comfortable with yoga, you can take turns suggesting a few poses. Otherwise, you can do some basic toe touching, and static lunging on one side and then the other. You can alternate stretching one arm across your chest and then the other, as well as interlacing your hands behind your back while you slowly bend over—so that your hands come up toward your head.

Most important, cheer each other on! Take a picture with your cell phone and share the joy with other friends, acknowledging a job well done. Maybe they'll want to join you next time too!

12

MOVE Your Brain

The phrase that had such a lasting impact on James has literally become gospel in our household: "All motion creates positive emotion." Exercise creates a cascade of chemical events that impact your brain, your body, and your emotions. Imagine dedicating yourself to something that will result in greater clarity, increased happiness, elevated moods, and decreased anxiety and depression. This link between depression and mood in relationship to exercise has actually been studied since the early 1900s. Even a single session of exercise can have a positive impact in individuals with a history of depression.[1] It is our opinion that choosing *not* to exercise is like choosing to be sad or depressed.

What keeps you from moving your body every day? What is your *but* that gets in the way of being at your best every day? What stories have you told yourself about why you don't need to make exercise a joyful and grateful priority in your life? Are you willing to open your mind and heart, and embrace exercise as one of the most powerful gifts you can give yourself every day to change your life?

Working Out and Working Within

Working out has come to mean many things, depending on who you ask. For some people, it may translate to an all-out sweat fest. For others, it may be a yoga session, a kickboxing class, lifting weights, swimming, biking, or martial arts. Working out generally means exerting a physical effort—moving the body in such a way that your heart, body, and mind reap the rewards of a job well done. Now, how many times have you heard someone say they have to work within or work in? We're guessing not too often.

Working within is when we take the necessary downtime to nurture our spirits. When we've been running around nonstop, for example, or we've had five days in a row of intense physical exercise, it may be a good time to work within. That is, take an hour or thirty minutes in your day to really unwind. This may come in the form of a massage or meditation. Perhaps it is restorative yoga, journaling, gardening, or chanting. Whatever you choose, working in can have tremendous emotional and physical benefits.

You can actually work out and work within at the same time. This happens when you combine physical exercise with something that has deep or powerful meaning for you, connecting it to your intrinsic motivators, as we discussed before. Say you are a runner, and you run not just for your health but because you want to be a role model, serving as an inspiration for your children. While you are running, you can connect to these intrinsic motivators. For example, you can dedicate your first mile to compassion for your coworker, who may be struggling with his or her relationship. You can dedicate the second mile to unconditional love and the connection you have with your children. And to round out your 5K, you can simply run in gratitude—being grateful for your legs, your lungs, your arms, your running shoes, whatever you are feeling.

Another piece of working within is simply acknowledging your body. When we pay attention to our bodies, we are less likely to become obese, because we have an increased awareness of our physical needs. When we ignore our bodies, we tend to ignore physical exercise and what crosses our lips in terms of food—or alcohol or tobacco or junk; we stop listening to the needs of our bodies. Working within is about listening to your body.

Another way to look at working within is looking at how movement (aka working out) affects what happens on the inside. When we exercise, we feel better on the inside, and connect to our bodies and spirits. Exercise helps us feel more at peace with ourselves.

We are giving you permission to work within. Some days you may just be too exhausted, drained, depleted, sore, or tired. If this is the case, work on your inner strength. Work on your mental fitness. Work on loving yourself more. Practice yoga poses that keep you grounded on the floor (i.e., laying down). Work on paying attention to and acknowledging your beautiful, strong body. *Affirm* your beautiful, strong body. Be grateful for the ways it has supported you in the past few days or weeks. And the next day, get ready to move your body once again with powerful physical activity.

. . . .

ACTION STEP

Choose in this moment a picture of yourself that inspires you. See yourself physically fit. Look deep into your being and see vitality and confidence. See and feel what is like to be that person who honors their self-care with impeccable discipline and commitment. Know that vision of you is within you right now and ready to be unleashed. Start with where you are. Get dressed to Move. See it to be it. When you see yourself dressed and ready, chances are you will follow through.

. . . .

Thriving Under the Influence of Exercise

Exercise changes your brain. It was fairly recent—only a few decades ago—that researchers discovered that exercise can actually generate new nerve cells in the brain. With early research done primarily on mice (and later, monkeys), researchers were able to conclude that moderate exercise improved alertness, attentiveness, and increased learning times.[2]

We have discussed BDNF several times now. (Remember brain-derived neurotrophic factor? It's the Miracle-Gro protein that's always ready to potentiate your good mood, your clarity, and your cognition.) When we are stressed (under the influence of high cortisol), BDNF decreases. When we exercise, BDNF increases! BDNF is critical to protecting your brain cells (neurons) from damage and death, and for helping them to grow and become stronger. For example, lower levels of circulating BDNF are an independent risk for increased mortality in older women (over eighty-five years).[3] But you have the power to create BDNF at every age with the right food, movement, and lifestyle.

Exercise is the ultimate smart pill! Movement sparks both physical and mental fitness. One particular study was done with students in Naperville, IL. This school community, like others across the country, was seeing a dramatic drop in math and science scores and overall performance. So someone decided they needed to make some changes and turn things around. What this school district did was awesome, and it has started a revolution. These pioneers created what is referred to as "Zero Hour PE," scheduled first thing in the morning, at 7:00 AM. This timing is strategic in that it happens just before math and science classes, which begin the school day. What has this move done for the students? Over the last dozen-plus years that Zero Hour PE has been in place, Naperville kids have been crushing their science and math scores. Their scores always rank in the top tier of the country. These kids who are moving every morning are fired up intellectually, emotionally, and physically. Their brains are firing and wiring at an optimum level, and they are happier and healthier too.[4]

Other studies have reported similar findings. Researchers at Michigan State University verified that students (two hundred sixth graders) who participated in vigorous sports did 10 percent better in science, English, math, and social studies compared to other students.[5] We are emphasizing vigorous here because students in the regular PE class did not do any better or worse in their academic classes, which is interesting. For us, that means if you are going to take the time to make exercise happen, make it count by really pushing yourself.

So what does it mean to Thrive under the influence of exercise? It means increasing BDNF levels through interval training, resistance training, and aerobic exercise. This improves our thinking, our mood, and our clarity. Thriving under the influence of exercise means pushing ourselves outside of the comfort zone yet paying attention to our body, listening to its needs.

Dr. James Reveals the Magic Pill
http://youtu.be/HaJs11XZN50

Mental Fitness

The healthiest brains are attached to bodies that move; regular, strong, and vigorous exercise strengthens circulation for body and mind. Exercise makes the brain more adaptable and higher functioning. One of the saddest and greatest tragedies we have witnessed as human beings and primary care providers is the devastating effects of Alzheimer's disease (AD). Alzheimer's disease is the sixth leading cause of death in the United States.[6] The loss of one's mind is cruel to the affected person, and their loved ones and caregivers are deeply affected as well. Treatment for AD and dementia is very challenging and costly. The latest statistics from the American Alzheimer's Association show that in 2013, an estimated 5.2 million Americans of all ages had AD. One in nine people age sixty-five and older has AD, and 32 percent of people age eighty-five and older have AD.[7]

In cultures around the world that exhibit the greatest longevity, it is rare to see dementia and Alzheimer's disease. Why? What is it that we are doing here in the United States that drives this disease and makes it so commonplace? Our Western way of eating and not moving are primary risk factors. Higher levels of physical activity are linked to a reduced risk of AD.[8] Prevention is our best opportunity to fight this growing trend.

The *Journal of Nutrition, Health and Aging* published a study that boasted the ability of exercise to protect our brains. The study showed that people with the highest level of activity were less likely to develop Alzheimer's disease compared to people who were inactive. Exercisers were also 50 percent less likely to develop any form of dementia or mental impairment.[9]

A study from the *Annals of Internal Medicine* found that older adults who exercised three or more times per week had a 30 to 40 percent lower risk for developing dementia than their more sedentary counterparts.[10] And in a review of studies published in the *Archives of Medical Research*, researchers concluded that there is indeed a "robust" association between physical activity and a reduction in memory impairment.[11] The message is simple and encouraging: the more we Move, the better we Think.

The hallmarks of a diseased brain are its rigid pathways and appearance—when the brain becomes hardened by lack of blood flow, increased inflammation, and lack of stimulation. In Alzheimer's disease, for example, the brain will usually have a large quantity of amyloid plaques and neurofibrillary tangles (these are types of protein fragments that cannot be dissolved). There is also a loss of connection between nerve cells. But exercise may help to help bridge those connections, possibly by rerouting neurons or creating new connections.[12] Think of exercise as a direct lifeline to mental fitness, along with cognitive and emotional resilience.

Move with Confidence

Exercise helps us feel better physically, which translates to feeling better mentally and emotionally. This gives us a greater sense of well-being, and translates to greater overall confidence and self-esteem. And since exercise helps relieve stress, it allows us to better manage challenges that come our way. When we overcome challenges, confidence increases. Exercise also increases the amount of oxygen flowing to the brain, which can stimulate greater clarity and confidence.

Your brain houses it's own pharmacy of chemicals that can either support or hinder confidence, motivation, and clarity. Remember those neurotransmitters we described earlier? Dopamine serves as a powerful catalyst to enliven and bring forth greater confidence. Exercise increases both your level of dopamine and the number of receptor sites, which allows for greater absorption. When under the influence of dopamine, you will be more likely to have higher levels of motivation, confidence, and conviction. Another cool side effect of having optimum levels of dopamine is that it may also help with curbing addictive behaviors to sugar, alcohol, cigarettes, and other challenging substances. And the best time to crank up your dopamine stores is first thing in the morning.

We've mentioned our propensity for morning movement. Our physiology is wonderfully vulnerable to building and releasing our chemical dream team (dopamine, serotonin, norepinephrine) first thing in the day. When we nourish our bodies with exercise first thing in the morning, we tend to have greater confidence, motivation, and resistance to addiction and sugar cravings all day long—and we're not talking about running a marathon every morning. Dopamine responds best to shorter exercise bouts at greater intensity (again, think HIIT).

• • • • • • • • • • • •

ACTION STEP

For the next week, commit to waking up just thirty to forty-five minutes earlier than usual and include exercise in your morning routine. (If you already have some time built into your mornings, simply commit to adding exercise.) Commit to writing in your journal immediately after exercising and around midmorning—at least a few words that explain how you feel adding this into your routine. We're willing to bet you'll feel inspired to continue the ritual, and then you'll be able to see it in writing: proof that including exercise in the morning feels wonderful!

• • • • • • • • • • • •

Exercise supports a healthier self-esteem and positive body image. And healthy self-esteem and self-confidence bring forth an entirely different energy into relationships, both personal and professional. It's fairly obvious when a person is confident or insecure. Sure, you can fake confidence, but wouldn't you rather experience the authentic feeling? Exercise supports that feeling, that healthy glow—that inner knowing that you have what it takes to persevere through life's ups and downs. You are unshakeable.

Exercise: Elevate Your Mind

What does Thriving look like to you in relationship to movement and exercise? Can you see how regular exercise stimulates your brain and your self-confidence? Write down four proactive steps you can take immediately to support your mental health. Maybe it is scheduling one day of downtime to focus on your inner wellness. Perhaps it is doing something physical that stretches you and helps build confidence. Follow through on your steps and continue to journal the experience.

Whether you are a busy mom, a surgeon, student, entrepreneur, financial planner, or unemployed, exercise will elevate your mental and emotional wellness to help you become the brilliant, kind, patient, and confident person that you were born to be.

We were all born for greatness; it's just that some of us forget it, as chronic adultness gets in the way. We're here to cheer you on to get started and to remind you to keep up the good work.

MOVE

Summary

Develop a positive body image.

- Consider what society tells you about what your body "should" look like and create the intention to love yourself right where you are.
- Look to your thoughts, eating habits, and exercise regime to judge your healthfulness, not your body type and weight.
- Remember that you can exercise every day and still carry extra weight.
- Just because you are "normal weight" or even underweight doesn't mean you are healthy.
- Love yourself no matter what your body size, and be inspired to make that body Thrive.

Stop with the excuses and start moving!

- Exercise is not just for your body; it is also for your mind, and can improve focus and mood.

- Dress the part: when you have the gear that helps you perform and feel your best, exercising will feel that much better and more enjoyable.
- Even if you don't have a lot of time, look into efficient workouts, like HIIT, to make the most of the time you do have.
- Take moments throughout your day to fit in incidental fitness whenever you can.

There are as many ways to Move as there are diets, so don't feel hindered by your options.

- Add high-intensity interval training (HIIT) to your exercise regime; it will up your GH levels and provide many antiaging benefits.
- Embrace building lean muscle by interspersing HIIT with strength training.
- Consider adding yoga to your fitness schedule to lengthen muscles, improve flexibility, improve mind–body benefits, and bring peace and calm to your life.
- Don't be afraid to mix it up by adding Zumba, Nia, tennis, swimming, dance, and so forth to your exercising to keep things fresh and keep you interested.

All movement creates positive emotion.

- When we exercise, BDNF increases, helping you grow your brain and mood.
- Exercise makes your brain more adaptable and higher functioning, as well as decreases the risk of Alzheimer's.
- Exercise gives us a greater sense of confidence and self-esteem.
- Don't just work out; work *within* by learning to be present in your body and mindful in every moment.

THRIVE

I celebrate myself, and sing myself.

—**Walt Whitman**

What does it mean to Thrive? Thriving is not a destination but a journey. It is moving beyond happiness, the absence of depression, a cute butt, a healthy pocketbook, or a cool car. To Thrive is to really know yourself—know your passions, your purpose, your deepest longings, your mission, and your vision for your life. When we are Thriving, we are on fire with purpose. We are being of service and making a difference in the world. We are nurturing our bodies and minds with impeccable self-care, positive thinking, healthy eating, and regular movement.

Thriving is all about excelling and going beyond self-imposed limits. Who are you when you inspire yourself and others? What are you doing? How are you carrying yourself? What kinds of thoughts are you thinking? What do you want the world to be? Are you willing to show up, and be that big and bold? Are you willing to be that powerful and loving?

Living, playing, and thriving affords us the honor of giving in an unlimited capacity. This is the place of serving up our *A* game, knowing that what we do, how we act, and the way we live has an effect on everything and everyone around us.

Thriving is when your actions are fueled by a love of high service, and the service is all heart, no ego—truly selfless. We transcend ourselves when our livingness serves to inspire greatness in others.

The world needs people to Thrive. So many people are sad, lonely, wired, tired, unhealthy, and disconnected from the truth of who they really are and what they came here to be. Have we settled for status quo? Is this the best we've got? Has our disillusionment with the system led us to disbelieve in ourselves?

Standing for a movement against mediocrity is going to test every fiber of your being. Standing for yourself and others is what you came to this life to do; it's why you are here. This is your time. You are here to Thrive.

We believe self-love and self-care are forms of social activism. When practiced in alignment with big thinking, healthy eating, and daily movement, you will Thrive. What we know to be true is that you are created for magnificence. Your mind and body are designed for expressing inspiring vitality, powerful thoughts, and courageous action. Your spirit reveals this amazingness through physical means of expression—arts, sciences, technology, friendship, kindness, love—that only we, as humans, can do. You serve nothing and no one when you play small.

Exercise: Your Legacy
As you begin to Thrive, inspiring yourself and those around you, take out your journal and write down your intentions in response to these questions:

- What is it that you will leave behind as your legacy?
- How will you be remembered—good energy, kindness, service, generosity, love?

We tend to think of and limit ourselves by defining *legacy* as something we leave behind after we die. But we can—and should—become top until later than we'd like to admit. Yet we still take time to nurture friendships, spend meaningful family time with our daughters, exercise daily, and put quality food on the table every day and night. Sure, we may have had a head start; we've made this our life's work. And we've learned a ton along the way—what works and what doesn't. We've done a lot of weeding out in our lives, and it hasn't always been easy.

We are asking you to take a leap of faith—to courageously step up and choose to apply these tools to support your innate wisdom. There is a positive vulnerability we all have: an openness to receive our highest expression. You have everything that you need to step into the void and take action. Think, Eat, Move, Thrive (TEMT) is a philosophy for living well, but it will only come alive when you choose to dedicate yourself to living it. Inspired self-care is the most powerful form of healthcare. Know that you are a healer; and with each move you make toward thinking big, eating well, and moving with passion, power, and gratitude every day, you raise your vibration and create a wave that moves everyone in your wake.

Thank you for choosing to be openly awesome. We are grateful for your willingness to live with your heart out loud and, as Gandhi said, "be the change you wish to see in the world."

We believe we all deserve to Thrive. It is never too late to create—or re-create—the life of your dreams. Reclaim your awesome life today.

In peace, love, and thriving,

living legacies. We leave a legacy whenever we spend time
and act from our truest purpose, our heart. Look at how y(
the questions and ask yourself if you are currently living
The practice of living your legacy right now deepens your c
ence and fulfills your life's vision. If you want to be more fo
aligned, and more open to making connections to the peopl
that mean the most to you, connect to the big *why* you have
Connect your legacy to your mission and your vision. Now,
journal again, and this time, define your *living* legacy:

• What can you do right in this moment to live your legacy?
• What do you need to let go of in order to fulfill and live th

If you want to be remembered for your kindness and ge
kind and generous every day. If you want to be remembere
and giving, spend time volunteering for a cause that speaks t(
time helping at the food bank; volunteer at a shelter (human
give blood. If you want to be remembered as a great mother (
a great one now. Do less criticizing and faultfinding, and be n
supportive, and patient. Spend time with friends and family. 1
cable care of yourself so that you have the energy and good h(
care of others. Seek out people that you have been meaning o1
connect with, and let them know what they mean to you.

We came to write this book because, in spite of the thousan
within the wellness category, something was missing. The
behind *Think Eat Move Thrive* is quite simple: when you attach
why, your mission and your vision, and practice the simple p
Think, Eat, and Move, you will indeed Thrive. When you crea
of peace, happiness, success, and harmony within yourself, it
others and spread throughout the world. And rest assured, we a
you to do anything that we don't do ourselves. We are busy pa
tors, and entrepreneurs that hit the ground running by 5:00 A1

living legacies. We leave a legacy whenever we spend time with others and act from our truest purpose, our heart. Look at how you answered the questions and ask yourself if you are currently living this legacy. The practice of living your legacy right now deepens your current presence and fulfills your life's vision. If you want to be more focused, more aligned, and more open to making connections to the people and things that mean the most to you, connect to the big *why* you have established. Connect your legacy to your mission and your vision. Now, get out that journal again, and this time, define your *living* legacy:

- What can you do right in this moment to live your legacy?
- What do you need to let go of in order to fulfill and live this legacy?

If you want to be remembered for your kindness and generosity, be kind and generous every day. If you want to be remembered as selfless and giving, spend time volunteering for a cause that speaks to you; spend time helping at the food bank; volunteer at a shelter (human or animal); give blood. If you want to be remembered as a great mother or father, be a great one now. Do less criticizing and faultfinding, and be more loving, supportive, and patient. Spend time with friends and family. Take impeccable care of yourself so that you have the energy and good health to take care of others. Seek out people that you have been meaning or wanting to connect with, and let them know what they mean to you.

We came to write this book because, in spite of the thousands of books within the wellness category, something was missing. The philosophy behind *Think Eat Move Thrive* is quite simple: when you attach your bigger *why*, your mission and your vision, and practice the simple principles of Think, Eat, and Move, you will indeed Thrive. When you create this level of peace, happiness, success, and harmony within yourself, it will touch others and spread throughout the world. And rest assured, we aren't telling you to do anything that we don't do ourselves. We are busy parents, doctors, and entrepreneurs that hit the ground running by 5:00 AM and don't stop until later than we'd like to admit. Yet we still take time to nurture friendships, spend meaningful family time with our daughters, exercise daily, and put quality food on the table every day and night. Sure, we may have had a head start; we've made this our life's work. And we've learned a ton along the way—what works and what doesn't. We've done a lot of weeding out in our lives, and it hasn't always been easy.

We are asking you to take a leap of faith—to courageously step up and choose to apply these tools to support your innate wisdom. There is a positive vulnerability we all have: an openness to receive our highest expression. You have everything that you need to step into the void and take action. Think, Eat, Move, Thrive (TEMT) is a philosophy for living well, but it will only come alive when you choose to dedicate yourself to living it. Inspired self-care is the most powerful form of healthcare. Know that you are a healer; and with each move you make toward thinking big, eating well, and moving with passion, power, and gratitude every day, you raise your vibration and create a wave that moves everyone in your wake.

Thank you for choosing to be openly awesome. We are grateful for your willingness to live with your heart out loud and, as Gandhi said, "be the change you wish to see in the world."

We believe we all deserve to Thrive. It is never too late to create—or re-create—the life of your dreams. Reclaim your awesome life today.

In peace, love, and thriving,

ACKNOWLEDGMENTS

We are in awe of the process that brought this book to life. Through a series of auspicious events and introductions, James met Richard Cohn, founder of Beyond Words Publishing, and his beautiful wife, Michele. Richard invited us to stop by Beyond Words while we were out in Oregon celebrating our twentieth wedding anniversary. Our visit turned into a three-hour meeting, where we met most of the team and shared our ideas for *Think Eat Move Thrive*. Thank you, Richard, for saying yes and for believing in us. We are grateful for everyone at Beyond Words—especially for Emily Han and Gretchen Stelter, and their editorial diligence, conscious contributions, and patience.

We have been abundantly blessed with an inspired and loving tribe and family that stand by our side, praying, cheering, affirming, loving, and supporting us at every stage of the journey. They've been our MasterMind partners, they've let us live with them when we had nowhere to go, and they've held the vision that *Think Eat Move Thrive* is what the world really needs when it comes to a revolution. Thank you, Scott Carlin—dear friend, partner, and coconspirator in the creation of awesome, and the vehicle through which James met Richard at the Sun Valley Wellness Festival. Thank you, Cynthia James, Carl Studna, Ken Ludwig, and Lisa Livingstone, Dr. Roger and Erica Teel, for your affirmative prayers, your friendship, and your belief. Thank you, Karen, David, Izzy, and Emmy Zucker, for opening your home to all of us during what should have been an incredibly stressful time and welcoming us as part of your family. Thank you, Diane and Bob Beale, for your continuous love and support. Thank you, Malcolm Aylett, friend and advisor, for your love, guidance, and support. Thank you to our beautiful, supportive, loving, understanding, and patient daughters—Dakota and Elli—who put up with a dad who travels almost every week and a mom who spends way too much time at the computer. We love you both and are so grateful for all that you have taught us. And thank you to Jean Houston for sharing her words of wisdom in our foreword.

Debra wishes to thank Karen Zucker, Sue Kunimune, Sheri Jacobs, Christina Kohlruss, Linda Hoffman, Carol Stearns, Seth and Stacey Smith Chernoff, and Tom and Dawn Terwilliger for their wisdom and unwavering, solid, and unconditional friendship—always there for inspiration, laughs, advice, love, prayer, and support. To Cynthia James, for all of these same qualities, and for being my Mental Equivalent for unlimited possibilities. And to Sarah Symons, for raising consciousness around the planet, and for empowering and educating survivors of slavery; I'm so grateful for you and your friendship. And to Diane Beale, whose passion for human rights, women, and children uplifts and inspires me to do more and be more. Brother Paul and sister Tracy, I love you and thank God for you in my life. And to my parents, Uncle How and Aunt Bun, cousins—I'm so blessed and so grateful. And to my beloved James, whose heart, passion, charisma, love, and complete dedication to Thriving each and every day inspires and moves me deeply; thank you, love.

James wishes to thank Scott and Laura Carlin, Bill and Bob Groux, Rod Gaston, Robin Sharma and Darren Hardy, J. Madden (my spiritual friend, brother, and mentor), Amy Keller, Rob Coleman, Danny Sims, Kenny

ACKNOWLEDGMENTS

Kefalas, Ken Ludwig, MasterMind partners, and brother and sister Carl Studna and Cynthia James. Seth and Stacey Smith Chernoff, Richard and Michele Cohn, Tom and Dawn Terwilliger, Christina Kohlruss—thank you for being cheerleaders, visionaries, and cocreators in the movement against mediocrity. Thank you to John Allen for your love, partnership, and serving for Optimum Wellness. And to Greg Stroh, Rob Schuham, Alex and Ana Bogusky—thank you for being my Skooper tribe! My amazing and lovely mom, Carol, and Papa Bob, thank you, Dad—I miss you. And my inspiring and beautiful sister, Tamara, and brother, Bryan—I love you, and I am deeply grateful for the light you are in my life; thank you for being openly awesome for the world to witness. Finally—and with the deepest gratitude and love—I thank you, Debra Jeanne, my one and only: thank you for always being brave and saying yes to growing our life and our love.

Ultimately, we want to acknowledge you, the reader, for taking this trust walk with us and with yourself. It is through your demonstration of the practices of Think Eat Move Thrive that our mission and vision will be fully realized. And for that we offer our most heartfelt and deep gratitude.

This is the kind of book that never feels completely finished; we have so much more to share. But wellness is organic in nature—we are always learning and evolving. Gratefully, technology allows us to continue to support you beyond this book. Please stay connected with us through our thinkeatmovethrive.com website.

APPENDIX A

The TEMT Program

We love cooking and eating awesome, healthy food; and the TEMT Program is all about eating well and fully enjoying the experience, from shopping to preparing to eating—it's all good! The program is built on powerful and inspiring principles of health and wellness.

- **Mediterranean-style eating:** TEMT's core concept is the same "clean and intuitive eating" inherent in the Mediterranean diet, which hundreds of studies show to be one of the most effective eating plans for preventing a variety of chronic diseases and promoting a high level of vitality and longevity. Rich in fiber, healthy fats, lean proteins, and metabolically supportive complex carbohydrates, the program is both easy to follow and fully delicious. And the Mediterranean style of eating is naturally rich in antioxidants, which have antiaging and disease-preventing benefits. Rich in a variety of colors, this diet thrives on a good rule of thumb: the broader the range of colors, the greater the antioxidant power. Focus on eating a rainbow of colors every day!

Our Favorite Rainbow Foods on the TEMT Program

Wild salmon and other wild-caught or responsibly farmed fish:
These contain healthy omega-3 fats, and are thought to help
protect against heart disease and other inflammatory diseases.
But you need to be careful about the type and amount of fish
you consume. It is now recommended that most of us limit our
fish intake to no more than twice a week due to mercury concerns. We are very concerned about the health of our oceans
and water sources—projections concerning the safety of our
waters may have us rethinking the fish strategy in the very near
future. We recommend you stay on top of the seafood watch
by visiting the Monterey Bay Aquarium's Seafood Watch at
seafoodwatch.org.

**Blueberries/cherries/raspberries/strawberries/pomegranates/
cranberries:** With very high antioxidant activity, these fruits
offer brain and memory protection and benefits.

Olive oil: Naturally anti-inflammatory and rich in antioxidants,
olive oil has been shown to help protect against heart disease
and cancer.

**Nuts and seeds (walnuts, pistachios, almonds, flax, chia, hemp,
sunflower, pumpkin):** These little powerhouses contain beneficial fats and fiber, which may help protect against heart
disease and inflammation.

**Whole grains (oats, whole wheat, barley, brown or black rice,
quinoa):** Help stabilize blood sugar and insulin—maybe even
protect against heart disease—by eating whole grains. Just pay
attention to portion control. For example, when eating oat-

meal, stick to one cup (cooked); and for brown rice, no more than a half-cup (cooked).

Red/purple grapes (red wine): Containing resveratrol, pycnogenol, and polyphenols (all said to prevent heart disease), grapes are both delicious and healthy. But grapes have high sugar content, so you don't want to go too crazy with them. Wine in moderation is the only way to go. No more than one glass a day for most of us; and for women with a family history of breast cancer, consider skipping the alcohol altogether, as alcohol consumption may increase your risk for breast cancer.

Garlic (onion, shallots): These flavorful beauties boast sulfur compounds that may protect against heart disease and some cancers.

Crucifers (broccoli, kale, cabbage, cauliflower, arugula): Indole alkaloids are key ingredients here, which may help to prevent cancer and other diseases. Crucifers are also high in fiber, antioxidant vitamins, and minerals. Eat lots of these dark-green leafies—lightly sautéed, roasted, steamed, and occasionally raw.

Tomatoes: Tomatoes aren't for everyone, but they do have some awesome nutrition for those who tolerate them well. Tomatoes contain lycopene, a powerful antioxidant shown to help stimulate the immune system and protect from certain cancers—especially prostate. Lycopene is more highly concentrated in cooked (canned) tomato products, including tomato paste, tomato sauce, and even ketchup.

Green tea: Rich in polyphenols, green tea may reduce the risk of heart disease, cancer, and stroke. Green tea also helps support a strong metabolism.

Bonus food: Dark chocolate! You can't go wrong with its flavonols (potent antioxidants). Plus, dark chocolate's very high on the happiness quotient, which could add years to your life on its own.

• **Meal frequency (MF):** With the TEMT Program you may be eating more often than you are accustomed to. Paramount to sustained energy, powerful metabolism, and overall well-being is to support the maintenance of balanced blood sugar and hormonal harmony. This is naturally achieved by following the TEMT meal plan, and by honoring your physiological needs of eating every two to three hours throughout the day.

• **Post-workout performance nutrition:** Your body is ready to put your fat-burning machinery into overdrive directly after you complete your workout. The key to making this happen is twofold: (1) Be sure to eat within thirty minutes of your workout, and (2) consume between 10 to 15 grams of protein and 10 to 30 grams of carbohydrates (depending on how long and hard you were exercising). This practice will help to ensure your muscles are adequately refueled for proper and healthful recovery. (Protein is necessary to repair and build the muscle that you just broke down.)

Quick Science/Physiology Lesson

Exercise creates something called catabolism, which simply means the breakdown of tissue. In order to get your body back into an anabolic state (ensuring that you are building lean muscle and burning fat), you need to fuel yourself appropriately. If you miss eating the right food within the right time, you will miss the most metabolically powerful time of your day—and your results will suffer.

- **Promoting your natural GH:** Growth hormone (GH) is a natural substance produced by the body that peaks in our teen years and slowly declines thereafter. Coupling its decline with unhealthy lifestyle habits (high stress, high sugar, lack of exercise, lack of quality sleep, imbalanced eating), we add insult to injury and fast-forward the aging process. TEMT is built to naturally support healthy hormone balance. Combined with the exercise principles we have outlined, you will help your body produce GH naturally and support your brain, body, and Spirit in Thriving, no matter what your age!

Each day, what we choose to eat is the key to how we look and feel. What we consume is essential to the prevention (or risk) of type 2 diabetes, heart disease, metabolic syndrome, obesity, and even certain cancers. Whenever we embark on a new adventure, we do our best to prepare ourselves for the journey. Get in the habit of planning your days and your meals in advance, so you decrease the possibility of added stress in the mornings and the need to shop every day.

If you are doing this program as an individual (meaning you are cooking for one and not as a couple, or for your family), most recipes can be cut in half or served as a half, with one portion saved for lunch or dinner the following day. We have tried to be mindful of cost, and therefore, if your favorite vegetable is on sale or you find a better price on certain produce, feel free to substitute according to our lists of preferred vegetables and fruits. We do recommend choosing organic produce (and meats) whenever possible, but we know this isn't an option for everyone. It's our belief that the health payoff is ultimately worth the initial expense, though availability may be the larger issue. For a list of the best nonorganic choices, refer back to chapter 7 and the Environmental Working Group's list of the Clean Fifteen.

Here are the general goals of TEMT that you can get started on right away:

- Begin your exercise program
- Eliminate refined sugars
- Eliminate white and refined flours
- Eliminate fried food
- No more drive-thrus
- Add plenty of dark-green leafy vegetables
- Drink fruit juice only in small doses and diluted (no more than 4 ounces a day—too much sugar) or skip it altogether (recommended)

The following table features what we like to call our preferred foods. In most cases, we have listed what one serving looks like. The exception would be eggs, which will vary according to individual taste and recipes prepared. We recommend no more than an average of six eggs a week, and that's being generous. In addition, as we said earlier, use organic options whenever possible.

Carbohydrates		
Sweet potatoes (½ cup)	Pitted prunes (6)	Broccoli (1 cup)
Quinoa (½ cup, cooked)	Bell peppers (1 cup, cooked or raw)	Zucchini (1 cup)
Apple (1 medium)	Whole-grain pasta (1 cup cooked)	Hummus
Greens (unlimited)	Brown rice or wild rice (½ cup, cooked)	Kale (1 cup cooked, 2 cups raw)
Carrots (1 cup, chopped)	Barley (½ cup, cooked)	Mango (½ medium)
Asparagus (1 cup)	Pear (1 medium)	Spinach (1 cup cooked, 2 cups raw)

Carbohydrates, cont'd		
Oats (not instant) (1 cup, cooked)	Cauliflower (1 cup)	Eggplant (1 cup)
Beans and legumes: black beans, garbanzo beans, lima beans, pinto beans, unsalted peanuts, adzuki beans, navy beans, soy beans (all ½ cup); lentils (¼ cup)	Plain lowfat or nonfat yogurt (6 ounces)	Cherries (10 large)
Berries (1 cup)	Grapefruit (½ medium)	Artichoke

Proteins*		
Free-range chicken or turkey breast	Grass-fed, lean, free-range beef	Wild salmon (4 to 5 ounces)
Buffalo	Eggs (max 6 per week)	Lowfat cottage cheese
Alaskan halibut	Mussels	Scallops
Lean cuts of pork or ham	Skim cheeses (1 ounce)	Chunk light tuna (water packed)
Whey or brown rice protein powder (2 tablespoons)	Tofu or tempeh	Edamame (½ cup)
Milk (skim, 1%, 2%; 1 cup)	Plain Greek-style yogurt (6 ounces)	Alaskan cod
Arctic char	Rainbow trout	Crab

*4 ounces, unless otherwise noted

Fats		
Olive oil (preferred)	Canola oil	Nuts and seeds: almonds, walnuts, macadamia, pecans, pistachios (¼ cup)
Flaxseed oil and seeds	Hempseeds	
Coconut oil	Avocado	

Basically, most vegetables are unlimited. Think kale, chard, spinach, broccoli, asparagus, artichoke, mixed greens (and lettuces) for salads, carrots, and celery.

A Day in the Life of TEMT

Upon rising: Hydrate, meditate, journal, exercise (within an hour of waking), breakfast (400–600 calories).9:00 AM: Hydrate. (You should have consumed at least [approximately] 20 ounces of water by now.)

Midmorning: Snack (150–300 calories). Take a five- to ten-minute time-out for mental health. Stretch. Take a walk. Practice lunging down the hallway, going up and down a few flights of stairs, or your favorite yoga pose.

Late morning: Hydration check. (You should be at around 40 ounces.)

Midday: Lunch (400–600 calories).

Early afternoon: Take another personal mental health time-out.

Mid–late afternoon: Snack (150–300 calories).

Late afternoon: How are you doing with water? (You should have fulfilled your minimum by now—remember half your body weight [but in ounces]).

Evening: Dinner (400–700 calories).
Total calorie intake: It should be around 1600–2500 calories, depending on your individual needs and goals.

Put this practice to work today and watch your mind, body, and emotional positivity become a force for ever-growing greatness!

Portions

Portion control is an essential component of TEMT. We recommend picking up a small kitchen scale (found at most grocery stores), which is helpful when you are starting out and getting used to recognizing proper portion sizes. The following list applies to an average meal.

- 3 to 4 ounces of meat, poultry, fish, or alternate protein (about the size of a woman's palm or a deck of playing cards)
- ½ cup of cut fruit, vegetables, or pasta (about the size of a small fist)
- 1 cup of milk, yogurt, or chopped greens (about the size of a small hand holding a tennis ball)
- 1 ounce of cheese (about the size of your thumb, or 4 dice)
- 1 ounce of nuts (about 25 peanuts, 17 almonds, or 5 walnuts)

Snacks

To keep your appetite in check, make sure your 100- to 300-calorie snacks contain a bit of protein, fiber, and fat, along with some carbohydrates. These kinds of balanced snacks—like peanut butter on a whole-grain cracker, for example, or an ounce of cheese with a pear—will satisfy your appetite as well as reduce the amount of food you'll eat at the meal that follows. Note: one nut is approximately 7 to 9 calories, so if you are eating large handfuls of nuts, the calories will add up quickly. Again, be mindful of portions.

In between your meals (which will hover roughly around 400 to 500 calories, or approximately 1200–1500 calories per day), will be two snacks. Aim for about 200 calories for each snack, and consider healthy alternatives to grab-and-go snack bars.

A Word About Snack Bars

There are so many bars on the market these days. Whether you are hardcore vegan, raw food enthusiast, or paleo crusader, there's a bar for you. Be watchful of calories, and read the labels closely; look at fiber content. Do not buy any bars that contain hydrogenated or partially hydrogenated oils, or high-fructose corn syrup. Ideally aim for bars around 200 calories or less unless you know you'll be skipping a meal; then a higher calorie bar may help until you can get your next real meal.

Snacks Around 100 Calories

- 1 piece of string cheese
- 1 cup of grapes
- 1 cup of strawberries
- 1 large apple
- 10 baby carrots with ¼ cup hummus
- An orange and 5 or 6 almonds
- 10 cashew nuts
- 10 almonds
- 2 ounces of lean roast beef or turkey
- Half of a small avocado
- 1 hard-boiled egg and half of a sliced cucumber
- ¼ cup of cooked brown rice, with 1 fresh tomato and ½ ounce of hard cheese
- 4 mini rice cakes, with 2 tablespoons of lowfat cottage cheese
- 3 ounces of lowfat cottage cheese and 3 whole-wheat crackers

- ¼ cup fat-free ranch dressing, with mixed raw veggies
- 1 small baked potato, with ½ cup salsa and 2 tablespoons of fat-free sour cream
- ⅓ cup of unsweetened applesauce with 1 slice of whole-wheat toast, cut into strips for dunking
- One 5-ounce tossed salad with lettuce, tomato, cucumber, and ¼ cup fat-free dressing
- 10 ounces of coconut water
- ¾ cup of cooked edamame
- One 8-ounce nonfat, soy, or almond milk latte (no flavor syrups or sugar added)

Snacks Around 200 Calories

- 25 almonds
- ¾ cup of strawberries with ½ cup of nonfat cottage cheese
- 4 ounces of grilled chicken
- Turkey-and-cheese roll-ups (144 calories): Cut 1 part-skim mozzarella cheese stick in half lengthwise. Roll about 1 ounce of sliced roasted turkey breast around one half of the cheese stick and repeat with the remaining cheese stick and another 1-ounce slice of turkey to make a total of two roll-ups.
- 3 ounces of deli turkey slices with 1 ounce of lowfat Cheddar cheese
- 1 apple with 1 tablespoon plus 1 teaspoon of peanut butter or almond butter
- 2 tablespoons of hummus with 2 rice cakes
- ½ cup slow-cooked oatmeal with ½ cup nonfat milk
- 2 ounces of Spence & Co. Wild Salmon Pinwheels (160 calories)
- 6 whole-grain or multi-seed gluten-free crackers with 2 teaspoons of nut butter or hummus
- 1 cup drinking coconut milk blended with 1 scoop sprouted brown rice protein powder plus ½ cup frozen berries.
- Half of a baked sweet potato (bonus when sprinkled with cinnamon)

- Half of a whole-wheat English muffin with 1 hard-boiled egg, sliced tomato, lettuce, and onion
- 1 small whole-wheat pita (4 inches in diameter) with ¼ cup of baba ghanoush
- 2 ounces of shrimp cocktail, with ¼ of an avocado and 1 tablespoon of cocktail sauce

 Dr. James's Favorite Snack
http://www.youtube.com/watch?v=z6Lst-Gv8YS4&list=PLDF26DC5254801299

Inflammatory and Anti-Inflammatory Foods

There has been a lot of research on which foods contribute to inflammation and which foods are anti-inflammatory, but one thing is certain: the food you eat has a direct impact on the inflammation in your body.

Inflammatory Foods

- Sugar, all types (white sugar, brown sugar, confectioners' sugar, corn syrup, processed corn fructose, turbinado sugar, etc.)
- Processed (refined) foods, including processed meats
- Junk food and most fast food
- Fried food (fried chicken, potato chips, french fries, etc.)
- Excess red meat and fatty meat
- Foods high in saturated fats
- Food additives
- White bread
- Ice cream
- Oils such as vegetable and corn (unless cold pressed)
- Trans-fat, hydrogenated and heated polyunsaturated oils
- Soda, caffeine, and alcohol
- Movie popcorn

Anti-inflammatory Foods

- Fresh whole fruits and vegetables
- Dark-green leafy vegetables
- Bright, multicolored vegetables
- Deep-sea, cold-water, low-mercury, oily fish
- Green tea
- Extra-virgin olive oil
- Nuts, legumes, and seeds, especially very fresh walnuts
- Low-glycemic-index foods
- Pure water (filtered water)
- Spices, especially turmeric, curry and ginger

APPENDIX B

Your Next 30 Days with TEMT

We're excited to share this program with you! It is a bit more detailed than the typical diet programs that you may have experienced in the past, but we have been creating successful programs like TEMT for the past ten years. In that time, we have had great feedback and success from individuals who first follow the plan and then adapt it to become a part of their normal lifestyle. That is our goal for you too: after thirty days of TEMT thinking, eating, and moving, you will have the tools you need to choose foods mindfully and wisely for the rest of your life.

We'll allow TEMT to speak for itself, but here are a few preliminary notes: Each day's menu averages around 1600 to 1800 calories, and an asterisk (*) next to any menu item indicates that the recipe is included at the end of the book. This calorie intake may not be enough for you if, for example, you are already an endurance or highly trained athlete, you are an active male, or you fall into a low BMI [body mass index] category. Please pay attention to what your body is telling you, using your best judgment to add calories as needed. And use fresh, sustainable (humanely raised) organic foods/ingredients whenever possible. As for the gratitude and movement exercises, they are, of course, optional. Feel free to substitute your workout of choice, and use your own journal for your daily gratitude practice.

A note on condiments: Be conservative; most condiments have added sugars (and high-fructose corn syrup). Aim for no more than ½ teaspoon mayonnaise and a few teaspoons each of ketchup and mustard on top of burgers or sandwiches. Also, try to use raw nuts whenever possible to avoid unnecessary sodium and potential trans (or unhealthy) fats.

• • • • • • • • • • • •

Day 1

Affirmation: *I am profoundly grateful for all of my successes—big and small!*

Today I am grateful for:

_____

Menu:
- Breakfast: Kale-Shallot Frittata*
- Snack: Plain Greek yogurt, ⅓ cup berries, 2 tablespoons granola
- Lunch: Broccoli Soup,* mixed-greens salad (optional), whole-grain roll
- Snack: 20 almonds, 1 apple
- Dinner: Honey-Lime Shrimp with Quinoa and Cucumber-Tomato Salad*

Exercise: Ten-minute jump-rope intervals. Do 1 minute jump rope, 30 seconds rest, 1 minute jump rope, 30 seconds rest—for 10 minutes.

Alternate jumping on both feet, hopping on one foot then switching; alternate speed and depth of knee bend. Follow this with 3 sets of 10 push-ups and 50 sit-ups.

• • • • • • • • • • • •

Day 2

Affirmation: *I am motivated by a deep connection to my personal worth and the value of the changes I am making!*

Today I am grateful for:

_____

Menu:
- Breakfast: Quinoa porridge (½ cup cooked quinoa, ½ teaspoon cinnamon, dash vanilla, 2 tablespoons lowfat milk or almond milk), ½ pear (sliced or diced), 1 tablespoon walnuts
- Snack: 1 apple (sliced), 1 tablespoon nut butter
- Lunch: Roasted Beet Salad with Chicken, Goat Cheese, and Walnuts*
- Snack: 2 slices natural, nitrite-free turkey breast, 10 whole-grain crackers or grain-free raw crackers
- Dinner: Lentil and Sweet Potato Stew*

Exercise: Wind sprints or speed-walking intervals. On a treadmill, track, or safe stretch of road or trail, warm up with a slow jog or walk for 5 minutes. Sprint or walk as fast as you can for 40 seconds, followed by 20 seconds of recovery (walk or slow walk), followed by 40 seconds of sprinting and a 20-second recovery. Do this for 5 cycles, then cool down with a jog or walk for 5 minutes. For a longer workout, add several sets of intervals. Follow up with 5 minutes of stretching or yoga.

• • • • • • • • • • • • •

Day 3

Affirmation: *I love my life, my mind, and my body. Every day I am more fit and healthy!*

Today I am grateful for:

_____

Menu:

- Breakfast: Dr. James's Grain-Free Pancakes* (made with almond meal/ flour)
- Snack: ½ red grapefruit
- Lunch: Chicken (or turkey) and wild rice soup (broth based; 12 ounces), whole-grain roll or crackers (optional) (Vegetarians can have broth-based bean or legume soup)
- Snack: ¼ cup hummus, 3 carrot sticks (or other raw veggies)
- Dinner: Baked sweet potato (small), 5 ounces baked (or grilled) wild salmon, fresh greens (steamed or lightly sautéed in olive oil: 1 to 2 cups spinach, kale, chard, cabbage, broccoli, or a mixture)

Exercise: Get outdoors. Take a hike, take the dog for an extra loop, go for a bike ride, ski, snowshoe, or paddle board (depending on the weather!).

• • • • • • • • • • • •

Day 4

Affirmation: *I am supercharged by my vision of a healthier, happier me!*

Today I am grateful for:

_____

Menu:
- Breakfast: Green Power Smoothie*
- Snack: Ants on a log (2 pieces celery with 1 tablespoon peanut butter spread on top and dotted by 1 tablespoon raisins)
- Lunch: Green Chickpea Salad*
- Snack: 1 hard-boiled egg; 1 small whole-grain pita (or slice of gluten-free bread); sliced tomato and onion; lettuce leaves
- Dinner: Stuffed Squash*

Exercise: Yoga class. Challenge yourself with a yoga class today. Either sign up online or go and check out your local recreation/yoga center, and get your down dog on!

•   •   •   •   •   •   •   •   •   •   •   •

Day 5

Affirmation: _I honor my body with the energy-giving vitality of exercise!_

Today I am grateful for:

_____

Menu:
- Breakfast: ½ cup steel-cut oats (cooked), 1 to 2 tablespoons chopped macadamia nuts, cinnamon, ½ banana
- Snack: 6 ounces plain Greek yogurt, ½ cup chopped pineapple (or berries), 1 teaspoon ground flaxseed

- Lunch: White Bean and Barley Soup*
- Snack: Turkey roll-ups (2 thin slices turkey rolled around thinly sliced bell pepper [about ½ bell pepper] and ½ cup baby spinach leaves)
- Dinner: 1 small baked sweet potato or 1 cup homemade (baked) sweet potato "fries," baked halibut (5 ounces), sautéed chard (using 1 tablespoon olive oil)

Exercise: *Get your Spin on.* Hop on your bike or a stationary bike and do 15 to 30 minutes of intervals (or sign up for a spin class). Alternate speed and resistance and you'll work up a great sweat. Follow it up with 15 minutes of weight work, focusing on the upper body (bicep curls, triceps kick backs, shoulder presses, shoulder raises).

• • • • • • • • • • • •

Day 6

Affirmation: *Peace and joy are part of my inherent nature. I allow peace and joy to spring forth abundantly from within!*

Today I am grateful for:

_____

Menu:
- Breakfast: 1 poached egg, 1 gluten-free waffle (or pancake), 1 cup greens (steamed)
- Snack: ½ ruby red grapefruit
- Lunch: 4 ounces cooked free-range chicken, 2 cups tossed mixed greens, unlimited raw veggies (Vegans can substitute chicken with grilled tofu, ½ cup garbanzo beans, or ½ cup edamame.)
- Snack: ½ cup lowfat cottage cheese, carrot and celery sticks

- Dinner: Roasted veggies (cauliflower, broccoli, squash—about ½ cup each), black bean tacos (2 corn tortillas; ½ cup beans [whole or lowfat refried]; ⅓ avocado, diced; 1 ounce lowfat mozzarella cheese [optional]; salsa; shredded cabbage)

Exercise: Core work. Warm up with a 10-minute bike, jog, or walk. Then alternate balancing on one foot then the other, while bringing opposite elbow to opposite knee. Do 3 sets of 15 reps (each side). Now lie on your back and perform this same bicycle movement (the exercise you just did standing, alternating elbows to knees). While still on your back, use your core muscles to lift your legs straight up above you, engaging your gut muscles as you lift your hips off the ground about 3 inches; then go back down to the ground (perform 3 sets of 15 reps). Follow this with 50 abdominal crunches or standard sit-ups. Roll over and come to a plank pose (like the beginning of a push-up). Time yourself to see how long you can hold the plank (aim for at least 1 minute). Rest for 30 seconds in between holds. Repeat 3 times. Follow with 3 sets of 15 push-ups.

• • • • • • • • • • • •

Day 7

Affirmation: *I am capable of and deserve greatness in every area of my life. I follow my bliss, and my life unfolds magnificently.*

Today I am grateful for:

_____

Menu:
- Breakfast: Strawberry-coconut smoothie (1 cup frozen strawberries, 6 ounces [unsweetened] almond milk or coconut water, 2 tablespoons

light coconut milk, 2 teaspoons shredded coconut, 1 scoop vanilla protein powder, 1 scoop powdered greens [optional; we always use Skoop, which you can purchase at drdeb.healthyskoop.com])
- Snack: ½ cup pumpkin seeds, 2 clementines (seedless tangerines)
- Lunch: Hummus or tuna fish wrap (3 tablespoons hummus or ⅓ cup tuna; 1 ounce lowfat cheese; one gluten-free tortilla [or 2 corn tortillas]; ½ teaspoon lowfat mayonnaise and mustard, as desired; ¼ cup spinach leaves, chopped; 1 roasted red pepper, chopped [about ¼ cup])
- Snack: Smoked salmon with goat cheese on crackers (You'll need ½ ounce spreadable goat cheese or soy cheese; ½ teaspoon fresh chopped dill; ¼ cucumber, sliced; 2 ounces smoked wild salmon; 5 rice or gluten-free crackers. Mix dill into spreadable cheese, spread 1 teaspoon on each cracker, top with a slice of cucumber and a piece of smoked salmon.)
- Dinner: Fava, Spinach, and Quinoa Cakes*

Exercise: Get scared. Physically challenge yourself with something that scares you. Whether it be swimming or dancing in public, get out of your comfort zone and thrive in the newness.

. . . .

Day 8

Affirmation: *My thoughts reflect the vision and mission I have for my life.*

Today I am grateful for:

_____

Menu:
- Breakfast: ½ cup muesli (unsweetened), 4 to 6 ounces almond milk (or nondairy milk of choice), 1 scoop protein powder (optional)

- Snack: 6 pieces vegetable sushi rolls (made with brown rice, avocado, cucumber, carrots)
- Lunch: Mixed field greens or spinach salad; 2 tablespoons dressing (or less); 4 ounces grilled, roasted, or baked protein of choice; 1 table-spoon pine nuts
- Snack: 1 pear, 1 lowfat string cheese
- Dinner: 5 ounces boneless, skinless chicken breast (marinated in lemon juice and olive oil, and sprinkled with your favorite dried herbs and spices), baked or grilled; 1 small baked sweet potato; 1 cup roasted Brussels sprouts (we love them drizzled with a little bit of olive oil and a dash of salt and pepper, and roasted at 375°F for 20 minutes) or other green vegetable of choice

Exercise: Boot camp. Create your own challenging regimen, look online for a workout, or head to your nearest recreation center or CrossFit gym.

• • • • • • • • • • • •

Day 9

Affirmation: *I consciously surround myself with people who raise me up.*

Today I am grateful for:

_____

Menu:
- Breakfast: Nutty brown rice or quinoa cereal (½ cup cooked brown rice or quinoa, 2 tablespoons chopped walnuts, 1 tablespoon ground flax, dash cinnamon, 1 to 2 tablespoons lowfat milk of choice, ½ grape-fruit, 1 teaspoon honey [optional], 1 to 2 tablespoons protein powder [optional])

- Snack: Green Smoothie* or berry smoothie of choice
- Lunch: Avocado, Quinoa, and Chicken Salad*
- Snack: 1 cup edamame
- Dinner: Italian turkey burger with mixed-greens salad and vinaigrette (To make turkey burger, mix ¼ pound ground turkey [per person], ½ cup finely chopped spinach, and ¼ teaspoon Italian herbs [a mix of oregano, basil, thyme, garlic, and parsley]. Add 1 teaspoon Parmesan cheese and mix together until spices and cheese are well incorporated. Grill indoors or out. Serve "naked" on top of a big mixed-greens salad or open face on a gluten-free bun or toast, with a slice of tomato and onion on top.) See note regarding condiments on page 216.

Exercise: Chop wood, carry water. This is a metaphor, of course, for get up, get outside, move naturally. Volunteer somewhere like Habitat for Humanity or the local food bank. Whether you are hammering nails, carrying boards, or moving cans, you'll be working and moving your body.

• • • • • • • • • • • •

Day 10

Affirmation: *I focus on my powerful* Why, *knowing that self-care is a form of social activism.*

Today I am grateful for:

_____

Menu:
- Breakfast: 2 poached eggs, 1 small bowl oatmeal (⅓ cup raw rolled oats), cinnamon, ½ ruby red grapefruit

- Snack: 1 cup raspberries
- Lunch: 1 cup of Black Bean Soup* (canned or see recipe), salad of mixed greens with 1 tablespoon vinaigrette
- Snack: 1 ounce almonds, 1 apple
- Dinner: Grilled wild salmon (4 to 5 ounces), sautéed veggies (1 teaspoon olive oil, unlimited greens), ½ cup cooked quinoa

Exercise: Box jumps. If you don't have a legitimate "plyometric" box, use a sturdy bench or step (the height should cater to your ability). We recommend starting out with something about knee high or, if you have knee issues, maybe 4 to 6 inches off the ground; and step up rather than jump. Execute 10 to 15 repeated jumps, rest for 30 seconds, and repeat 3 to 5 times. Follow up with 3 sets of 25 jumping jacks, 3 sets of 10 to 15 push-ups, and 5 minutes of stretching.

• • • • • • • • • • •

Day 11

Affirmation: *As I take care of myself, I am able to give more and grow more. I am a blessing to the world.*

Today I am grateful for:

_____

Menu:
- Breakfast: Green Smoothie II*
- Snack: ½ cup homemade gorp (5 almonds, 5 walnuts, 2 Brazil nuts, 3 macadamia nuts, 10 raisins, 10 dark chocolate chips)
- Lunch: Cobb Salad*

- Snack: ½ cup lowfat cottage cheese, 6 rice crackers (optional: drizzle with ½ teaspoon honey)
- Dinner: Mediterranean Lemon Chicken with Dill and Vegetable Rice*

Exercise: Break free. Get outside for a hike.

• • • • • • • • • • • •

Day 12

Affirmation: *I am grateful for all my successes, however great or small.*

Today I am grateful for:

_____

Menu:
- Breakfast: Vegetable scramble (2 eggs [or substitute 1 cup tempeh], ½ cup chopped veggies of choice, 1 tablespoon lowfat goat cheese or shredded mozzarella [optional])
- Snack: ½ cup granola, ½ cup almond milk or 6 ounces plain Greek yogurt
- Lunch: Chopped Greek Salad with Chicken*
- Snack: 10 slices cucumber, 1 to 2 tablespoons lowfat ricotta (or marscapone cheese), 2 tablespoons dried, chopped apricots (Mix the ricotta with the apricots to make a spread.)
- Dinner: Sweet Potato Turkey Tacos with Black Beans*; 1 cup kale, steamed or sautéed in no more than 2 tablespoons of olive oil.

Exercise: Music for your moves. Create a new playlist of your favorite songs to sweat to. Then take them for a test walk/run to see if you're really feeling it.

. . . .

Day 13

Affirmation: *I am motivated by my desire to serve and live life as a high performer and mentor to those around me.*

Today I am grateful for:

_____

Menu:
- Breakfast: ½ cup cooked quinoa with cinnamon (optional: stir in 1 scoop whey/rice protein), ½ cup berries, almond milk (or lowfat milk), 1 tablespoon chopped pecans
- Snack: 6 ounces plain yogurt, ½ cup sliced strawberries, 1 teaspoon ground flax
- Lunch: Tuscan-Style Tuna Salad* over bed of mixed greens, 6 whole-grain crackers (optional)
- Snack: 2 mandarin oranges (Cuties) or 1 regular orange, 1 lowfat string cheese
- Dinner: Acorn Squash Stuffed with Chard and White Beans*

Exercise: Wind sprints. See Day 2.

. . . .

Day 14

Affirmation: *I stay alert to my resistance and limiting moods. I call forth deeper, intrinsic inspiration and motivation, and allow it to guide me!*

Today I am grateful for:

_____

Menu:
- Breakfast: Huevos Rancheros Verdes*
- Snack: Blueberry smoothie (⅓ cup frozen blueberries; 6 ounces water, almond/lowfat milk, or coconut water; 1 scoop protein powder; 1 scoop greens [optional]; 5 fresh or frozen strawberries [optional])
- Lunch: Simple macrobiotic plate—⅓ cup black beans; ½ cup cooked brown rice; 1 cup steamed broccoli (and/or other green veggies of choice, or cauliflower); 1 tablespoon sunflower seeds; a few tablespoons soaked hijiki or arame seaweed (optional); ¼ avocado, diced; wheat-free (gluten-free) tamari soy sauce, Bragg's liquid aminos (a tablespoon or less), and dulse (a seaweed)—all to taste (all optional)
- Snack: 1 apple or pear, 1 tablespoon nut butter
- Dinner: 5 ounces grilled halibut with Mango-Avocado Salsa,* ½ cup cooked brown or black rice, 2 cups spinach or chard, sautéed (in 1 teaspoon olive oil)

Exercise: Move with your neighbors. Get involved in the community. Sign up for a movement class or community-supported event like a 5K.

• • • • • • • • • • • • •

Day 15

Affirmation: *The nurturing of my mind and body is a celebration of my life!*

Today I am grateful for:

_____

Menu:

- Breakfast: ½ cup cooked steel-cut oats; 2 tablespoons chopped macadamia nuts; dash cinnamon; ½ banana, sliced
  (To make steel-cut oats, note that they take about 40 to 60 minutes to cook. Add about 3 cups of water to 1 cup steel-cut oats, bring to a boil, lower heat, cover, and simmer until water is absorbed and oats reach desired consistency [you may need to add more liquid]. This recipe makes 3 cups, so you will have 6 servings. You can freeze a partial batch if desired, but the cooked steel-cut oats should keep for about 5 days in the refrigerator.)
- Snack: ½ cup fresh berries, ½ cup cottage cheese
- Lunch: 1 cup lentil soup (homemade or canned [low sodium]), sautéed greens (kale, spinach, chard, and/or collards in 1 tablespoon olive oil with, 1 tablespoon sliced almonds and 1 garlic clove)
- Snack: Raw veggies—1 carrot (chopped into sticks), 1 stalk celery, ½ red bell pepper, ¼ cup hummus or baba ghanoush
- Dinner: Pork Tenderloin with Blueberry Sauce*; ½ cup cooked brown rice; 10 asparagus spears, steamed or sautéed (in ½ teaspoon olive oil)

Exercise: Intervals. Choose jump-roping, mountain climbers, burpees, push-ups, or jumping jacks; grab your stopwatch; turn up your playlist; and get moving! Aim for about 20 minutes of intervals (10 cycles of 30 seconds on, 30 seconds off).

• • • • • • • • • • • •

Day 16

Affirmation: *Beyond a destination, I embrace thriving as a joyous way of being!*

Today I am grateful for:

_____

Menu:
- Breakfast: Dr. James's Grain-Free Pancakes* (made with almond meal/flour)
- Snack: 1 pear with either 1 lowfat string cheese, 1 tablespoon nut butter, or 15 almonds
- Lunch: Turkey Cheddar apple wrap (You'll need 3 to 4 thin slices deli turkey [about 2 ounces], 1 teaspoon mustard, or to taste [we like spicy mustard]; 1 slice [about 1 ounce] lowfat Cheddar cheese; 2 to 3 lettuce leaves; ⅓ medium Granny Smith apple, thinly sliced; 1 sprouted-whole-grain or gluten-free tortilla. Spread mustard on tortilla; layer with turkey, cheese, apple, and lettuce [or save apple for the side]).
- Snack: 1 sliced cucumber, 1 ounce spreadable cheese (Laughing Cow, goat, or cream cheese), 1 ounce smoked wild salmon
- Dinner: ½ cup cooked quinoa; ⅓ cup cooked pinto beans; steamed vegetables of choice (generous amount); 1 ounce shredded cheese, if desired; salsa (a simple but delicious meal)

Exercise: Lower-body strength training. Begin with 5-minute warm-up (either walking, biking, or elliptical trainer). Then 3 sets of 15 repetitions each: lunges with medium weights (add bicep curls with each lunge as a bonus), squats, leg extensions (these are easiest when you have a weight bench and weighted plates; but if you don't have that, you can sit on the edge of a chair or bench, strap a small weighted tote around your ankle, and lift from there), hamstring curls, side leg raises.

• • • • • • • • • • • •

Day 17

Affirmation: My body responds effortlessly to the vision of wholeness I give it!

Today I am grateful for:

_____

Menu:
- Breakfast: 2 poached eggs (or 3 pieces of tempeh [3 ounces]; ½ cup cooked brown rice (roughly ¼ cup uncooked); 1 handful baby spinach (about a cup), sautéed (in 1 teaspoon olive oil)
- Snack: ¼ cup pumpkin seeds, 2 dates
- Lunch: Tuna Caesar salad (2 cups romaine lettuce, torn into bite-sized pieces; 1 tablespoon Caesar dressing; 1 tablespoon crumbled feta or shredded Parmesan cheese; 2 ounces canned tuna [in water]; ¼ avocado, sliced; 10 whole-grain or gluten-free crackers)
- Snack: 1 cup kale chips (homemade or store bought)
- Dinner: Easy Chicken Parmesan*; 1 cup steamed broccoli; ½ cup cooked brown rice, quinoa, or brown-rice pasta (optional)

Exercise: Out and about. Get outdoors for an energizing hike or brisk walk.

. . . .

Day 18

Affirmation: *I connect with and identify my passion and purpose for a healthy and thriving lifestyle!*

Today I am grateful for:

_____

Menu:

- Breakfast: ½ cup unsweetened muesli with 6 ounces Greek yogurt or ¾ cup organic milk, almond milk, or organic soy milk
- Snack: 1 celery stalk, 1 tablespoon peanut butter (or nut butter of choice), ½ cup strawberries
- Lunch: White Bean and Barley Soup*
- Snack: Turkey and cheese roll-ups (1 to 2 ounces [1 to 2 slices] natural, nitrite/nitrate-free turkey breast or ham, 1 lowfat string cheese [Cut cheese in half and wrap each with a piece/slice of meat].)
- Dinner: 5-ounce piece Pacific flounder (sole), cod, or other white fish (To prepare fish, squeeze about a tablespoon of fresh lemon juice; drizzle a teaspoon of olive oil; and sprinkle dried or fresh herbs of choice [about ¼ teaspoon], such as rosemary or thyme, on top of fish; then bake at 400°F for about 15 minutes, until fish is cooked through and flakes easily with a fork); 1 small baked potato (or sweet potato) with skin; 1 cup steamed or sautéed greens of choice (drizzled with 1 teaspoon extra-virgin olive oil [EVOO])

Exercise: Yoga. Take a break to breathe, stretch, and center yourself for 30 minutes to an hour.

• • • • • • • • • • • •

Day 19

Affirmation: _All of my efforts are enhanced by an attitude of positivity, peace, ease, and grace._

Today I am grateful for:

_____

Menu:
- Breakfast: Veggie scramble, ½ ruby red grapefruit (In a medium-sized skillet coated with cooking oil spray or 1 teaspoon unsalted butter, add ½ cup chopped veggies of choice, 1 to 2 eggs [or ¼ cup tempeh or tofu], 1 tablespoon lowfat goat cheese or shredded mozzarella [optional]. Cook until veggies are soft and eggs are set.)
- Snack: 12 pistachios, ½ cup fresh (or ¼ cup dried) blueberries
- Lunch: Arugula greens (generous amount); 4 ounces cooked chicken (or tofu), 1 tablespoon pine nuts, 1 tablespoon feta (or goat cheese), 1 tablespoon balsamic vinaigrette or vinaigrette of choice, 1 sliced fresh fig (if in season)
- Snack: Smoked salmon with goat cheese on crackers (You'll need ½ ounce spreadable cheese; ½ teaspoon chopped dill; ¼ cucumber, sliced; 2 ounces smoked wild salmon; 8 rice or gluten-free crackers. Mix dill into spreadable cheese and spread 1 teaspoon on each cracker. Top with a slice of cucumber and a piece of smoked salmon. Alternatively, skip the crackers and load everything on top of cucumber slices.)
- Dinner: "Naked" burrito (½ cup cooked brown rice; ½ cup cooked black beans; 3 ounces cooked chicken or pork [optional]; ¼ avocado, diced; 2 tablespoons salsa; ½ to 1 ounce shredded cheese of choice [lowfat]; shredded romaine lettuce [as much as you wish]; diced cilantro, to taste; lime juice, to taste [optional]; 1 dollop plain Greek yogurt, in place of sour cream [optional])

Exercise: Interval swimming. Head to your nearest lake or pool. Warm up with easy, freestyle swimming for 5 minutes. Then alternate strokes and speeds for 20 minutes. Rest when needed. You should feel your heart beating. Stretch in the water or on dry land for 5 minutes after your intervals.

• • • • • • • • • • • •

Day 20

Affirmation: *I am thriving daily. I celebrate my healthy and beautiful body!*

Today I am grateful for:

_____

Menu:
- Breakfast: 6 ounces plain Greek yogurt (lowfat), 2 tablespoons walnuts, ¼ cup berries, dash cinnamon
- Snack: 10 cashews, ½ ounce dark chocolate
- Lunch: Chicken Salad with Olive Vinaigrette*
- Snack: Endive with ricotta and cranberries (Take 4 endive leaves and place 1 tablespoon part-skim ricotta on each leaf. For a hint of sweetness, sprinkle 2 tablespoons dried cranberries over the ricotta.)
- Dinner: Curry Grilled Salmon,* ½ cup cooked brown rice, 1 cup roasted cauliflower (To roast, drizzle the cauliflower with a light coating of extra-virgin olive oil and roast in the oven at 375°F for 15 minutes)

Exercise: Cardio dance party. Either put on your favorite tunes at home or head to your nearest Zumba or Nia class. Or, if you are so inclined, sign up for tango or swing dance lessons, and get your groove on that way.

• • • • • • • • • • • • •

Day 21

Affirmation: *I am on purpose with my healthy thinking, eating, and moving; and I Thrive in every area of my life.*

Today I am grateful for:

_____

Menu:
- Breakfast: Green Power Smoothie*
- Snack: ¾ cup raspberries (fresh or frozen), ½ cup lowfat cottage cheese
- Lunch: 4 ounces grilled (or cooked) shrimp on 2 cups mixed greens, ½ cup chopped mango, 1 tablespoon favorite dressing
- Snack: 1 cup tomato soup, ½ whole-grain roll or ½ slice whole-grain or gluten-free bread (optional)
- Dinner: Chicken fajitas (You will need 4 ounces chicken, ½ red bell pepper [chopped], ½ green bell pepper [chopped], and ¼ onion, cut into slivers. Use fajita spice mixture [cumin, chili powder, garlic powder, dash cayenne, and smoked paprika] and stir-fry or sauté the chicken and veggies until chicken is cooked through. Serve "naked" over ¼ cup pinto beans or black beans and ½ cup cooked brown rice; and top with 2 tablespoons lowfat shredded cheese of choice, 1 tablespoon nonfat sour cream [or plain Greek yogurt], and ¼ avocado [sliced]. Accompany with a side salad of mixed greens [2 cups] with vinaigrette of choice).

Exercise: Wind sprints. See Day 2.

• • • • • • • • • • • • •

Day 22

Affirmation: *I believe in myself and move through challenges with confidence and zeal!*

Today I am grateful for:

_____

Menu:
- Breakfast: 1 cup favorite gluten-free, whole-grain cereal or ½ cup low-sugar, high fiber granola; ¼ cup nuts or dried fruit; ¾ cup almond milk or lowfat milk. (Optional: add a scoop of protein powder to your milk and blend it before adding to your cereal.)
- Snack: 1 cup seasonal fresh fruit, 2 tablespoons raw nuts or seeds
- Lunch: Salmon niçoise salad (You will need 3 or 4 torn romaine lettuce leaves; ½ can of wild [boneless, skinless] salmon; ¼ cup artichoke hearts; 5 black olives; 1 hard-boiled egg, sliced [optional]; 1 teaspoon capers; ½ cup diced tomato; 2 anchovies [optional]. Layer the ingredients as desired, and dress with 1 tablespoon olive oil and lemon juice [plus a dash of salt and pepper] or niçoise dressing
- Snack: 1 ounce lowfat string cheese or cheese of choice, 1 kiwi
- Dinner: Stuffed Peppers*

Exercise: Core work. See Day 6.

• • • • • • • • • • • •

Day 23

Affirmation: *I am impeccable with my words. I treat myself and others with kindness and nonjudgment.*

Today I am grateful for:

_____

Menu:
- Breakfast: Strawberry smoothie (½ cup fresh or frozen strawberries, 1 cup almond milk or lowfat milk, 1 teaspoon ground flax, 1 teaspoon chia seeds, 1 scoop protein powder, 1 tablespoon plain yogurt, ½ banana)
- Snack: ½ to ¾ cup cooked oatmeal, 1 tablespoon ground flax, dash cinnamon, ½ cup diced apple
- Lunch: Power Ranch Salad*
- Snack: 2 carrot sticks, 2 stalks celery, 2 tablespoons hummus
- Dinner: Thai chicken (or tofu) stir-fry over quinoa (Chop 3 ounces boneless, skinless chicken breast [or tofu] into bite-sized cubes; mince ½ teaspoon fresh ginger; chop 2 scallions, ½ red bell pepper, ½ zucchini. Using 1 teaspoon olive oil, stir-fry chicken, ginger, and scallions until chicken is almost cooked through. Add red bell pepper and zucchini, and continue to stir-fry. Add ½ teaspoon curry powder and ¼ teaspoon garlic powder [or add fresh minced garlic—about 1 clove], plus 1 teaspoon tamari soy sauce and ½ teaspoon fish sauce [optional]. Continue to sauté until chicken is fully cooked and veggies are tender. Serve over ½ cup cooked quinoa [or brown rice]).

Exercise: Mother Nature workout. Get outdoors and break a sweat: biking, intervals, hiking—your choice.

• • • • • • • • • • • • •

Day 24

Affirmation: *I commit to personal excellence. I give 100 percent to every meaningful area of my life, starting with my own self-care.*

Today I am grateful for:

_____

Menu:
- Breakfast: Two-egg scramble, ½ ruby red grapefruit (You will need 1 egg plus 1 egg white, 1 cup chopped spinach, dash salt and pepper, 2 tablespoons salsa [optional]. Scramble all ingredients together in a nonstick skillet [or coat skillet with olive oil or cooking oil spray] until eggs are cooked through)
- Snack: ½ cup plain Greek yogurt (lowfat), 1 tablespoon shredded coconut (unsweetened), ¼ cup fresh berries
- Lunch: Quinoa and Black Bean Salad,* 3 ounces grilled or baked chicken breast
- Snack: 2 carrot sticks, 2 stalks celery, ¼ cup hummus
- Dinner: Arugula Salad with Scallops and Basil*

Exercise: Two-part workout. Do yoga or stretching for at least 30 minutes in the morning, then take a 15-minute walk or jog midday.

• • • • • • • • • • • • •

Day 25

Affirmation: *I believe in the power of my body to transform, heal, be powerful, and be blessed with vitality and radiant health.*

Today I am grateful for:

_____

Menu:
- Breakfast: ½ cup steel-cut oatmeal, 2 tablespoons chopped macadamia nuts, dash cinnamon, ½ cup berries
- Snack: 1 apple, 10 raw almonds
- Lunch: Lentil salad (½ cup canned or cooked lentils; ½ cup chopped kale [sautéed with 1 teaspoon olive oil]; ¼ avocado, sliced; 2 slices tomato)
- Snack: (Humanely raised) turkey, chicken, or ham roll-ups (You'll need 2 slices roasted turkey breast with 1 slice provolone cheese divided in half [for each slice of turkey]. Roll up the meat and cheese, and enjoy with 10 baby carrots. Vegans can substitute 1 brown-rice cake with 2 tablespoons hummus of choice.)
- Dinner: 5 ounces boneless, skinless chicken breast (marinated in lemon juice and olive oil, sprinkled with herbs, baked until cooked through [350°F for about 25 minutes], 1 small baked sweet potato, 1 cup roasted Brussels sprouts or other green vegetable of choice

Exercise: Upper-body workout. See Day 5.

•   •   •   •   •   •   •   •   •   •   •   •

Day 26

Affirmation: *I am here for greatness!*

Today I am grateful for:

_____

Menu:
- Breakfast: Breakfast parfait (Layer 6 ounces lowfat, plain Greek yogurt with ½ cup sliced mixed berries [frozen or fresh], 2 tablespoons chopped walnuts, and ⅓ cup high-quality or homemade granola.)
- Snack: 2 mandarin oranges (Cuties) or 1 orange, 1 piece lowfat string cheese
- Lunch: 3 cups Kale Salad*
- Snack: ¼ cup hummus, 10 gluten-free crackers, 1 carrot (cut into sticks), 1 stalk celery
- Dinner: Grilled Mussels with Basil*; ½ cup cooked brown rice; 1 cup green beans, steamed or sautéed (in 1 tablespoon olive oil or 2 teaspoons unsalted butter).

Exercise: Give tennis a try. Most recreation centers or tennis centers have racquets that you can borrow. Sign up for a cardio tennis class, and you'll work up a great sweat as you improve your game. If you already play, challenge your fitness with a singles match or a cardio tennis clinic.

• • • • • • • • • • • •

Day 27

Affirmation: *This is my time to shine, pure and simple. I look for opportunities to shine my light in the world.*

Today I am grateful for:

_____

Menu:
- Breakfast: 2 poached eggs, sautéed greens (kale, broccoli, chard, and/ or spinach in 1 teaspoon olive oil), 2 tablespoons roasted tomatoes (for extra flavor)
- Snack: Green smoothie II*
- Lunch: Cobb Salad*
- Snack: 20 pistachios
- Dinner: Chicken and veggie stir-fry. (Add 2 teaspoons olive oil to a large, nonstick skillet and sauté 4 ounces sliced chicken breast until nearly cooked through. Add 1 cup broccoli florets; ½ red bell pepper, sliced; ¼ cup chopped shallot; 1 tablespoon wheat-free tamari soy sauce; 1 teaspoon low-sodium teriyaki sauce; and any desired spices. Continue sautéing until chicken is done. Serve with ½ cup cooked brown rice [measure after cooking] [Alternative protein: use diced, firm tofu or (peeled and deveined) shrimp.])

Exercise: Lower-body workout. See Day 16.

• • • • • • • • • • • •

Day 28

Affirmation: _I create windows of opportunity to move naturally throughout my day._

Today I am grateful for:

_____

Menu:

- Breakfast: 1 cup slow-cooked or steel-cut oatmeal, measured after it has been cooked (usually it is ⅓ cup uncooked); 1 tablespoon chopped or ground walnuts (or sliced almonds); ½ cup blueberries
- Snack: 6 ounces nonfat yogurt, 1 kiwi
- Lunch: Green Chickpea Salad*
- Snack: 1 string cheese, ½ Granny Smith apple
- Dinner: Turkey burger with sautéed mushrooms and onions; baked sweet potato; mixed-greens or baby-spinach salad with 1 tablespoon dressing of choice. (Slice 10 button or shiitake mushrooms into quarters and ½ red onion into slivers. Sautée in 1 tablespoon olive oil with a dash salt and pepper, and a splash white cooking wine [optional]; cook until soft.)

Exercise: Get outdoors. Hike or bike, or bundle up and snowshoe or ski.

• • • • • • • • • • • • •

Day 29

Affirmation: *Today and every day, I do my best. I am a work in progress, and I aim high to Thrive.*

Today I am grateful for:

_____

Menu:

- Breakfast: 2 slices whole-grain (or gluten-free) toast, ½ cup berries, ½ cup lowfat cottage cheese
- Snack: Green Power Smoothie*

- Lunch: Power Ranch Salad*
- Snack: ½ red bell pepper, sliced; 1 lowfat string cheese
- Dinner: Ginger chicken stir-fry (for one); ½ cup cooked quinoa or brown rice penne pasta (Cut 4 ounces boneless, skinless chicken breast into small, 1-inch pieces and set aside. Combine 1 tablespoon sesame oil, ¼ cup chopped onion, 1 clove garlic, and 1 tablespoon fresh minced ginger in a wok or large skillet; heat 2 to 3 minutes on medium high; add chicken; and cook until almost cooked through. Add ½ cup chopped green cabbage,½ cup chopped or sliced zucchini, and a little water or broth; and simmer until chicken is fully cooked and veggies tender).

Exercise: Boot camp. See Day 8.

• • • • • • • • • • • •

Day 30

Affirmation: *I am courageous, confident, and willing to evolve my life from average to amazing!*

Today I am grateful for:

_____

Menu:
- Breakfast: Huevos Rancheros Verdes*
- Snack: 1 sliced apple, dash cinnamon, 1 tablespoon almond butter
- Lunch: Cobb Salad*
- Snack: 1 cup black bean soup or tomato soup, 1 whole-grain roll, mixed-greens salad (about 1 to 2 cups with 1 to 2 tablespoons vinaigrette)

- Dinner: Honey Mustard Wild Salmon,* ½ cup cooked brown or wild rice (or substitute 1 small baked sweet potato), 1 cup steamed or sautéed greens of choice

Exercise: Work within today. Reflect on the past month; check in with yourself. Have you been adding movement to your daily life where it may have been lacking? Are you cutting down on the number of hours spent in front of the television? Journal your experience, and spend time in quiet meditation. Exercise your heart with a loving kindness meditation.

APPENDIX C

Recipes

Note: the recipes are listed in alphabetical order, not by category.

In general, with all of our recipes, we recommend the use of organic fruits and vegetables, dairy products, eggs, and humanely raised meats whenever possible. All grains, especially quinoa, should be thoroughly rinsed prior to cooking. When a recipe calls for olive oil, we recommend extra-virgin olive oil (EVOO). When a recipe calls for salt, we prefer sea salt. When a recipe calls for broth, we recommend low-sodium (or homemade). When we use anything like deli meat or bacon (turkey or pork) we always recommend you make sure it is nitrate and nitrite-free.

•   •   •   •   •   •   •   •   •   •   •   •

Acorn Squash Stuffed with Chard and White Beans

Serves 4
2 medium acorn squash, halved and seeded
1 teaspoon plus 2 tablespoons extra-virgin olive oil, divided

½ teaspoon salt, divided

½ teaspoon freshly ground pepper, divided

½ cup chopped onion

2 garlic cloves, minced

2 Tablespoons water

1 Tablespoon tomato paste

8 cups chopped chard leaves (about 1 large bunch)

1 15-ounce can white beans, rinsed

¼ cup chopped kalamata olives

⅓ cup finely chopped walnuts

⅓ cup grated Parmesan cheese

Position oven rack in center of oven and preheat to 375°F. Cut a small slice off the bottom of each squash half so it rests flat. Brush the insides with 1 teaspoon oil; sprinkle with ¼ teaspoon salt and ¼ teaspoon pepper. Place in a 9-by-13-inch (or similar size) baking dish. Cover with foil and cook for about 35 minutes or until tender. Remove from oven and raise temperature to broil.

Heat 1 tablespoon oil in a large skillet over medium heat. Add onion and cook, stirring, until starting to brown (2 to 3 minutes). Add garlic and cook, stirring, for 1 minute. Stir in the water, tomato paste, chard, and remaining ¼ teaspoon each salt and pepper. Cover and cook until chard is tender, 3 to 5 minutes. Stir in white beans and olives; cook until heated through, 1 to 2 minutes more. Remove from heat.

Spoon about ¾ cup to 1 cup of the chard mixture into each squash half; set aside.

Combine the walnuts, Parmesan, and remaining 1 tablespoon oil in a small bowl. Sprinkle squash with the Parmesan mixture. Place in the center of the oven until the top begins to brown, just a few (2 to 3) minutes.

Serve each squash in a shallow bowl, if there is extra stuffing you can serve that around the squash, or just add to the mound in the center of the squash.

Per Serving (½ stuffed squash): 474 Calories; 19g Fat (3g Sat.); 21g Protein; 61g Carbohydrate; 13g Dietary Fiber; 5mg Cholesterol; 828mg Sodium.

• • • • • • • • • • • •

Arugula Salad with Scallops and Basil

Serves 4
4 Tablespoons extra-virgin olive oil, divided
1½ Tablespoons fresh lemon juice
1½ Tablespoons balsamic vinegar
2 teaspoons grainy or Dijon mustard
1 teaspoon sugar or honey
½ teaspoon sea salt, divided
10 cups arugula
1 cup chopped basil leaves
½ cup roasted, chopped tomatoes
1 pound large scallops
¼ cup grated Asiago cheese
Freshly ground pepper

Whisk 3 tablespoons oil with the lemon juice, vinegar, mustard, sugar, and ¼ teaspoon salt in a small bowl; set aside.

Combine arugula, basil, and tomatoes in a large bowl; set aside.

Sprinkle scallops with remaining salt. Heat remaining tablespoon of oil in a large, nonstick skillet over medium-high heat. Add scallops and cook, turning or tossing from time to time, just until slightly browned on both sides and opaque in the center (2 to 3 minutes). (Alternatively, you can grill the scallops.)

Meanwhile, whisk the dressing again and pour over arugula mixture. Toss to coat, then divide salad mixture onto four plates.

Add scallops to the top of each salad and sprinkle with a tablespoon of cheese on each salad. Grind on pepper to taste, and serve while still warm.

Per Serving: 420 Calories; 19g Fat (3g Sat.); 31g Protein; 40g Carbohydrate; 8g Dietary Fiber; 44mg Cholesterol; 753mg Sodium.

• • • • • • • • • • • • •

Avocado, Quinoa, and Chicken Salad

Serves 4
1 cup uncooked quinoa, rinsed and drained
3 Tablespoons extra-virgin olive oil, divided
1 cup cooked, cubed chicken breast
1 small broccoli crown cut into bite-size florets
¼ cup diced yellow or red bell peppers
1 Tablespoon lemon juice
¼ teaspoon sea salt
¼ teaspoon freshly ground black pepper
½ avocado, peeled and diced
Fresh mint (4 sprigs), optional

Combine quinoa with 2 cups of water in a medium-sized pot and bring to a boil. Stir, reduce heat to low, cover, and cook for 15 minutes. Remove from heat (but keep covered).

Heat 1 tablespoon olive oil in a large skillet. Add chicken and stir-fry until just cooked through. Remove chicken from skillet, place in a small bowl and cover with a clean towel or foil. Return skillet to stove, add 1 tablespoon olive oil, and heat over medium heat. Add broccoli and red bell pepper and stir-fry over medium heat for about 5 minutes. Lower heat, return chicken to skillet, add cooked quinoa, and stir to combine. Set aside.

To prepare dressing, whisk together remaining 1 tablespoon olive oil, lemon juice, salt, and pepper in a medium bowl. Toss quinoa, chicken, and vegetable mixture with dressing, then gently stir in avocado.

Refrigerate until ready to serve. Serve in bowls garnished with fresh mint sprigs.

Per Serving: 404 Calories; 21g Fat (4g Sat.); 22g Protein; 33g Carbohydrate; 4g Dietary Fiber; 42mg Cholesterol; 215mg Sodium.

•   •   •   •   •   •   •   •   •   •   •

Black Bean Soup

Serves 8 to 10
1 pound dried black beans, soaked in water overnight and drained
4 quarts low-sodium vegetable broth or water
2 bay leaves
½ teaspoon dried thyme
½ teaspoon freshly ground black pepper
1 Tablespoon extra-virgin olive oil
½ cup diced onion
2 garlic cloves, minced
¼ cup diced green chiles
1 Tablespoon seeded and minced jalapeño pepper
1 teaspoon ground cumin
1 teaspoon ground coriander
1 teaspoon dried oregano
Salt and pepper
Lime wedges, to garnish
Cilantro sprigs, to garnish
Plain Greek yogurt, optional (½ cup)

Combine the beans and broth in a large soup pot and bring to a simmer. Add the bay leaves, thyme, and pepper. Simmer the beans, uncovered, approximately 2½ to 3½ hours. The beans should be very soft, just beginning to fall apart. Add additional broth if necessary.

Meanwhile, heat oil over medium heat in a small skillet. Add onion, garlic, green chiles, and jalapeño pepper; sauté for about 5 minutes, until onions soften. Add cumin, coriander, and oregano to this mixture and stir until well mixed.

Transfer ½ the beans and ½ the onion mixture to a blender and puree, adding water if necessary. Stir this mixture back into the remaining soup. Season to taste with salt and pepper.

To serve, garnish each bowl of soup with lime wedges and chopped cilantro and top with a dollop of yogurt if desired.

Per Serving: 322 Calories; 9g Fat (1g Sat.); 11g Protein; 45g Carbohydrate; 9g Dietary Fiber; 0mg Cholesterol; 1656mg Sodium.

• • • • • • • • • • • •

Broccoli Soup

Serves 6

2 cups water

1½ pounds broccoli (florets and about 2 inches of stalk), chopped

1 large stalk celery, chopped (¾ cup)

½ cup shredded carrots

1 medium onion, chopped (½ cup)

½ cup rolled oats

2 Tablespoons butter

2 Tablespoons potato flour or 1 tablespoon cornstarch (mixed in 1 tablespoon cool water)

2½ cups low-sodium chicken broth or vegetable broth

½ teaspoon salt
⅛ teaspoon pepper
Dash of ground nutmeg
½ cup lowfat milk or soy milk

Heat water to boiling in 3-quart saucepan. Add broccoli, celery, carrots, onion, and oats. Cover and return to a low boil. Simmer for about 10 minutes, or until broccoli is tender (do not drain).

Carefully place broccoli mixture in blender or food processor. Cover and blend on medium speed until smooth. Set aside.

Melt the butter in the same 3-quart saucepan over medium-low heat. Stir in flour mixture and cook, stirring constantly, until smooth and bubbly; remove from heat.

Stir the broth into the butter-flour mixture and return to the stove. At medium-low again, heat to boiling, stirring constantly for one minute.

Reduce heat; stir in blender contents; and season with salt, pepper, and nutmeg. Return soup to a low simmer, and stir in milk—do not boil. Turn off heat or keep on low until ready to serve.

Per Serving: 185 Calories; 12g Fat (4g sat); 6g Protein; 14g Carbohydrate; 4g Dietary Fiber; 27mg Cholesterol; 579mg Sodium.

•　•　•　•　•　•　•　•　•　•　•

Chicken Salad with Olive Vinaigrette

Serves 4
1 cup uncooked quinoa (or brown rice)
2 cups low-sodium chicken or vegetable broth
¼ cup pitted, chopped kalamata olives
2 Tablespoons chopped flat-leaf parsley

1 Tablespoon chopped capers

2 Tablespoons extra-virgin olive oil

1 Tablespoon fresh lemon juice

¼ teaspoon salt

¼ teaspoon freshly ground black pepper

1 garlic clove, minced

12 ounces cooked chicken breast, cubed and cooled

Rinse quinoa well. Combine with broth in medium-sized pot and bring to a boil. Reduce heat and cover for 15 minutes. Fluff with a fork, cover, and remove from heat for use later.

Combine olives, parsley, capers, olive oil, lemon juice, salt, pepper, and garlic in a large bowl, stirring with a whisk. Add quinoa and toss gently to coat. Toss in chicken just before serving.

Per Serving: 422 Calories; 19g Fat (3g Sat.); 32g Protein; 32g Carbohydrate; 3g Dietary Fiber; 58mg Cholesterol; 706mg Sodium.

•   •   •   •   •   •   •   •   •   •   •   •   •

Chopped Greek Salad with Chicken

Serves 4

⅓ cup red-wine vinegar

2 Tablespoons extra-virgin olive oil

1 Tablespoon chopped dill or oregano (or 1 teaspoon dried)

1 teaspoon garlic powder

¼ teaspoon salt

¼ teaspoon freshly ground pepper

6 cups chopped romaine lettuce

2½ cups chopped cooked chicken (about 12 ounces)

2 medium tomatoes, chopped

1 medium cucumber, peeled, seeded, and chopped
½ cup finely chopped red onion
½ cup sliced black olives
½ cup crumbled feta cheese

Whisk vinegar, oil, dill, garlic powder, salt, and pepper in a large bowl. Add lettuce, chicken, tomatoes, cucumber, onion, olives, and cheese; toss to coat, and serve.

Per Serving: 343 Calories; 18g Fat (5g Sat.); 31g Protein; 11g Carbohydrates; 3g Dietary Fiber; 89mg Cholesterol; 619mg Sodium.

• • • • • • • • • • • •

Cobb Salad

Serves 4
3 Tablespoons white-wine vinegar
2 Tablespoons finely minced shallot
1 Tablespoon Dijon mustard
1 teaspoon freshly ground pepper
¼ teaspoon salt
3 Tablespoons extra-virgin olive oil
10 cups mixed salad greens
8 ounces shredded cooked chicken breast
2 large eggs, hard boiled, peeled, and chopped
2 medium tomatoes, diced
1 large cucumber, seeded and sliced
1 avocado, peeled, pitted, and diced
2 slices cooked bacon (turkey or pork), crumbled
½ cup crumbled blue cheese (optional)

Whisk vinegar, shallot, mustard, pepper, and salt in a small bowl to combine. Whisk in oil until combined; set aside. Place salad greens in a large bowl, then add half of the dressing. Toss to coat. Divide the greens among 4 plates. Arrange equal portions of chicken, egg, tomatoes, cucumber, avocado, bacon, and blue cheese (if using) on top of the salad greens on each plate. Drizzle the salads with remaining dressing or serve on the side.

Per Serving: 352 Calories; 24g Fat (4g Sat.); 21g Protein; 18g Carbohydrates; 8g Dietary Fiber; 134mg Cholesterol; 445mg Sodium.

•　•　•　•　•　•　•　•　•　•　•　•

Curry Grilled Salmon

Serves 4

2 Tablespoons plain Greek yogurt
1 teaspoon lemon juice
2 teaspoons curry powder
½ teaspoon turmeric
½ teaspoon lemon pepper
¼ teaspoon salt
¼ teaspoon garlic powder
1 small shallot, diced
1¼ pounds wild salmon fillets, pin bones removed

In a small bowl, whisk together yogurt, lemon juice, curry powder, turmeric, lemon pepper, salt, garlic powder, and shallot. Set aside.

Place salmon in a shallow bowl and spread yogurt mixture evenly over each fillet (about 1 tablespoon per fillet). Cover and refrigerate for 30 minutes to an hour.

Heat grill to medium high (or heat oven to 425°F, or broil).

Place salmon on clean, greased grill or on a piece of aluminum foil placed directly on the grill, skin side down. Cook for about 10 minutes per inch of thickness, or until salmon is opaque and flakes easily when tested with a fork. Alternatively, bake in oven for 15 minutes, or until desired doneness is achieved.

This salmon is delicious served atop a bed of sautéed greens, quinoa, or brown rice.

Per Serving: 177 Calories; 5g Fat (1g Sat.); 29g Protein; 2g Carbohydrate; trace Dietary Fiber; 74mg Cholesterol; 276mg Sodium.

•　•　•　•　•　•　•　•　•　•　•

Dr. James's Grain-Free Pancakes

These are heavy-duty pancakes. You may want to eat one in the morning and save one for a snack a little later.

Makes two 5-inch pancakes (1 serving)
½ cup almond meal (aka almond flour)
2 eggs
1 to 2 Tablespoons ground flax (and/or chia seed)
½ teaspoon baking powder
1 to 2 teaspoons cinnamon
1 serving whey protein or your preference (James often uses brown rice protein)
Cooking oil spray
Fresh blueberries (small handful) (for the batter and/or to serve, optional)
1 Tablespoon Greek yogurt, jam, or pure maple syrup, to serve (optional)

In a medium bowl, stir or whisk all of the ingredients together until smooth. Ladle one pancake onto a medium-hot griddle lightly coated with cooking oil spray. Cook about 2 to 3 minutes on each side until golden brown. Repeat for the second pancake.

Serve warm with a side of Greek yogurt, berries, jam, or just a smidgen of pure maple syrup.

Per Serving: 531 Calories; 18g Fat (4g Sat.); 58g Protein; 22g Carbohydrate; 5g Dietary Fiber; 424mg Cholesterol; 542mg Sodium.

 Dr. James Cooks Up His Grain-Free Pancakes
http://www.youtube.com/watch?v=1gO8-rwzeDc&list=PLDF26DC5254801299

• • • • • • • • • • • •

Easy Chicken Parmesan

Serves 4
4 boneless, skinless chicken breasts, about 5 ounces each
½ cup rice flour (or almond meal)
¾ cup shredded Parmesan cheese
1 Tablespoon chopped oregano
1 egg
⅛ teaspoon salt
2 Tablespoons extra-virgin olive oil
Cooking oil spray
½ cup marinara sauce (Add up to 1 cup marinara if you desire a more saucy version)
½ cup shredded lowfat mozzarella cheese

Place chicken breasts (flat side down) on a sheet of plastic wrap and cover with another sheet of plastic wrap. Using a small saucepan, a rolling pin, or a meat tenderizer, carefully pound breasts to about ⅓-inch thickness. Pat breasts dry with paper towel and set aside.

In a small bowl, combine flour, Parmesan cheese, and oregano. In another small bowl, whisk together egg and salt. Brush both sides of the chicken breasts with egg, then lightly coat with the flour mixture.

Preheat oven to 400°F.

Warm the oil in a large, heavy skillet over medium-high heat. When oil shimmers, add chicken and cook about 3 minutes per side, until golden brown and cooked through. Transfer chicken to glass baking dish coated with cooking oil spray. Add 2 tablespoons (or more if desired) of marinara on top of each breast and sprinkle mozzarella evenly on top of each chicken breasts. Place chicken in oven for about 5 minutes or until cheese has melted.

Serve immediately. This is delicious on top of whole grain or gluten-free noodles, or with a side of brown rice.

Per Serving: 433 Calories; 18g Fat (6g Sat.); 46g Protein; 20g Carbohydrate; 1g Dietary Fiber; 155mg Cholesterol; 659mg Sodium.

•   •   •   •   •   •   •   •   •   •   •

Fava, Spinach, and Quinoa Cakes

Serves 4 to 6

20 ounces frozen chopped spinach, thawed
2½ cups fresh or frozen fava beans, thawed
4½ cups cooked quinoa
6 medium garlic cloves, minced
1 teaspoon salt, plus more to taste

1 teaspoon ground cumin
1 teaspoon ground coriander
½ teaspoon smoked paprika
½ teaspoon ground turmeric
4 egg whites
Black pepper
Preheat oven to 400°F.

Squeeze out as much water as possible from the spinach and set aside in a large mixing bowl.

Bring a medium pot of water to a boil (add a dash of salt while it is heating up). Add the fava beans and cook for 3 minutes. Drain, then pulse the beans in a food processor until a coarse puree forms. Add to the mixing bowl with the spinach.

Stir the quinoa, garlic, salt, cumin, coriander, paprika, and turmeric into the spinach mix. Add the egg whites and stir until well combined. Season with pepper and more salt as desired.

Form the mixture into 12 to 14 patties and place the patties on a parchment-lined baking sheet. Bake for 20 minutes, then flip and bake for another 5 minutes.

Serve on top a bed of fresh or sautéed greens. We especially like them on top of arugula drizzled with a bit of olive oil and a squeeze of lemon.

Per Serving (2 to 3 patties): 315 Calories; 3g Fat (trace Sat.); 22g Protein; 54g Carbohydrate; 17g Dietary Fiber; 0mg Cholesterol; 433mg Sodium.

.   .   .   .

Green Chickpea Salad

Serves 2
½ small jalapeño, seeded and finely diced (optional)
2 Tablespoons lemon juice
2 Tablespoons extra-virgin olive oil, divided
Salt and pepper
½ can chickpeas (about 1 cup), drained
½ bunch kale, spinach, or chard (enough for 2 to 3 cups shredded)
¼ cup shredded Parmesan

In a small bowl, combine jalapeño (if using) with the lemon juice and 1 tablespoon olive oil. Season as desired with salt and pepper. Add chickpeas, toss, and set aside.

Remove kale leaves from the stem and slice the leaves very finely, into shreds. Massage the remaining olive oil into the kale for about a minute.

Add the kale and Parmesan to the chickpeas, toss until well mixed.

Per Serving: 271 Calories; 11.5g Fat (2g Sat.); 12g Protein; 32g Carbohydrate; 9g Dietary Fiber; 4mg Cholesterol; 153mg Sodium.

. . . .

Green Power Smoothie

This is a go-to breakfast or snack of ours. Feel free to experiment with the ingredients until you find the green combination that is perfect for your palate.

Serves 1

6 to 8 ounces almond milk (we prefer homemade or plain unsweetened), coconut milk, or coconut water

½ cup coarsely chopped kale (4 ounces; well rinsed, stems removed,
firmly packed [baby kale works great])

½ Granny Smith apple, coarsely chopped (optional)

½ ripe banana, peeled and halved (optional; we like to freeze ripe
bananas for a thicker smoothie)

¼ avocado, peeled and sliced

1 Tablespoon plain Greek yogurt (or coconut yogurt)

1 scoop protein powder (we prefer vanilla whey protein or sprouted
brown-rice protein)

1 scoop powdered greens (try Skoop, formulated by Dr. James him-
self [available at drdeb.healthyskoop.com])

1 teaspoon almond butter (optional; good for when you desire a
super-charged, highly caloric smoothie)

Combine all ingredients in a blender and blend until smooth. If the mixture is too thick, add a little water. Serve in a chilled glass or mug.

Per Serving: 340 Calories; 9g Fat (2g Sat.); 29g Protein, 39g Carbohydrate; 8g Dietary Fiber; 1mg Cholesterol; 195mg Sodium.

. . . .

Green Smoothie II

Serves 1

6 ounces coconut water

1 Tablespoon almond butter

½ small cucumber, peeled

¼ medium apple, diced (with peel on)

2 Tablespoons chopped parsley

½ cup chopped kale

1 Tablespoon coconut milk

1 Tablespoon Greek yogurt

1 scoop sprouted rice protein (approximately 2 Tablespoons)

Combine all ingredients in a blender and blend until smooth. Drink right away.

Per Serving: 275 Calories; 8g Fat (4g Sat.); 30g Protein, 25g Carbohydrate; 6g Dietary Fiber, 1mg Cholesterol; 75mg Sodium.

. . . .

Grilled Mussels with Basil

Serves 4

1 pound fresh mussels

¼ cup fresh lemon juice, divided

2 Tablespoons unsalted butter, melted

½ cup dry white wine

Dash of hot sauce

¼ teaspoon dried crushed red pepper

¼ teaspoon dried basil

1 garlic clove, minced

Dash of salt

Dash of freshly ground black pepper

2 Tablespoons coarsely chopped basil, to serve

Remove the beards on the mussels and scrub the shells well with a brush. Discard open or cracked mussels; set the rest aside.

In a large bowl, combine 2 tablespoons of lemon juice with the melted butter, white wine, hot sauce, crushed red pepper, basil, and garlic; set aside.

Sprinkle mussels with salt, black pepper, and 1 tablespoon lemon juice; and place them in a grill basket.

Grill, over high heat (400° to 500°F), with the lid closed, about 10 minutes, or until shells open. Discard any unopened mussels.

Add mussels to the lemon mixture and toss well. Drizzle with remaining tablespoon lemon juice, and sprinkle with fresh basil. Serve immediately.

Per Serving: 174 Calories; 8g Fat (4g Sat.); 14g Protein; 6g Carbohydrate; trace Dietary Fiber; 47mg Cholesterol; 398mg Sodium.

• • • • • • • • • • • •

Honey-Lime Shrimp with Quinoa and Cucumber-Tomato Salad

Serves 4

1 Tablespoon extra-virgin olive oil

½ teaspoon black pepper, divided

Dash of cayenne pepper

Dash of salt
2 cucumbers, peeled and chopped
12 grape tomatoes, cut in half
1 lime, juiced
3 Tablespoons honey
3 Tablespoons grapeseed oil
¼ teaspoon salt
1 pound shrimp, peeled, tails removed, rinsed, and patted dry
2 cups cooked quinoa (from 1 cup raw)

In a medium bowl, combine the olive oil with ¼ teaspoon black pepper, cayenne pepper, and salt. Toss with the cucumber and tomatoes, and chill until ready to serve.

Combine lime juice, honey, grapeseed oil, salt, and ¼ teaspoon black pepper in a sealed glass container. Shake well, until thoroughly combined (it should look cloudy and smooth).

In a medium bowl, toss the shrimp with the lime juice marinade.

Heat a medium pan over high heat. When hot, pour in shrimp and marinade, and stir to prevent burning. Lower heat and cook for 3–4 minutes, until shrimp are opaque.

Transfer the shrimp (not the marinade) to a serving bowl, and cover to retain heat.

Add the quinoa to the remaining marinade in the pan and stir to combine over low heat. (The quinoa will soak up the flavor of liquid.) Heat until just warm, then set aside.

Serve shrimp on top of ½ cup quinoa on each plate, with cucumber-tomato salad on the side.

Per Serving: 446 Calories; 16g Fat (2g Sat.); 29g Protein; 43g Carbohydrate; 4g Dietary Fiber; 173mg Cholesterol; 312mg Sodium.

• • • • • • • • • • • •

Honey Mustard Wild Salmon

Serves 4

1½ Tablespoons Dijon mustard
1 Tablespoon lowfat ricotta cheese
2 Tablespoons chopped cilantro
2 teaspoons honey
1 to 1¼ pounds wild salmon, cut into 4 fillets (4 to 5 ounces each),
    pin bones removed
Dash of salt and black pepper

Preheat oven to 425°F.

In a small bowl, mix together the Dijon, ricotta, cilantro, and honey.

Place the salmon in a baking dish lined with foil, and spread the honey-mustard mixture on top of each fillet. Bake in the oven for 12 to 15 minutes, or until cooked through to the desired level.

Season with salt and black pepper, and serve warm. This dish goes well with most grains or a side salad of fresh arugula.

Per Serving: 269 Calories; 12g Fat (2g Sat.); 36g Protein; 4g Carbohydrate; trace Dietary Fiber; 97mg Cholesterol; 167mg Sodium.

• • • • • • • • • • • •

Huevos Rancheros Verdes

Serves 4

1½ cups finely shredded romaine lettuce
1 scallion, sliced

2 Tablespoons chopped cilantro

3 teaspoons canola or grapeseed oil, divided

2 teaspoons lime juice

¼ teaspoon salt, divided

¼ teaspoon freshly ground pepper, divided

One 15-ounce can pinto beans, rinsed

½ cup prepared green salsa (we love the 505 Southwestern brand)

Eight 6-inch corn tortillas

Canola oil cooking spray

3/4 cup shredded sharp Cheddar cheese

4 large eggs

Preheat oven to 400°F.

Combine lettuce, scallion, cilantro, 1 teaspoon oil, lime juice, ⅛ teaspoon salt and ⅛ teaspoon pepper in a medium bowl; set aside.

Combine beans and salsa in another medium bowl, and set this aside as well.

Coat both sides of each tortilla with cooking spray. Place the tortillas on a large baking sheet in 4 sets of overlapping pairs. (Each pair should overlap by about 3 inches.) Spread about ⅓ cup of the bean mixture on top of each pair of tortillas and sprinkle with 3 tablespoons cheese each. Bake until the beans are hot and the cheese is melted, about 10 minutes.

Heat the remaining 2 teaspoons of oil in a large nonstick skillet over medium heat. Crack each egg into a small bowl and slip them one at a time into the skillet, taking care not to break the yolks. Cook as desired, either over easy or sunny side up. Season the eggs with the remaining salt and pepper, or as desired. Reduce heat to medium low and cook undisturbed for 5 to 7 minutes for soft-set yolks. (For hard-set yolks, cover the pan after 5 minutes and continue cooking until the yolks are cooked through, 2 to 4 minutes more.)

To serve, place an egg on top of each pair of tortillas and top with a generous ¼ cup of the lettuce mixture.

Per Serving: 396 Calories; 18g Fat (6g Sat.); 20g Protein; 42g Carbohydrates; 8g Dietary Fiber; 234mg Cholesterol; 563mg Sodium.

• • • • • • • • • • • •

Kale Salad

Serves 4 to 6
1 bunch curly kale (about 10 cups when chopped into strips)
3 Tablespoons extra-virgin olive oil
1 small garlic clove, minced
Salt and pepper
2 Tablespoons fresh lemon juice
1 medium avocado, peeled and diced
2 medium scallions, thinly sliced
½ medium red bell pepper, diced
1 medium carrot, shredded or thinly sliced
2 Tablespoons pine nuts
2 Tablespoons chopped cilantro
1 Tablespoon chopped mint

Wash and dry the kale, and remove the leaves from the thick stem. Chop the leaves into thin strips and place in a large bowl. Add olive oil, garlic, salt, and pepper; massage into the kale until it is well coated. Add the lemon juice and continue to massage into the greens for about 1 minute. (Massaging the kale is actually really essential to tenderizing the kale and cutting its bitter flavor.)

Add the avocado, scallions, pepper, carrot, pine nuts, cilantro, and mint to the bowl and toss until all are well distributed throughout the salad. This is a great dish to bring to a potluck or family gathering.

Per Serving (based on 4 servings): 221 Calories; 20g Fat (3g Sat.); 3g Protein; 10g Carbohydrate; 3g Dietary Fiber; 0mg Cholesterol; 21mg Sodium.

Dr. James on Kale
http://www.youtube.com/watch?v=WzMi-aXqHVs&list=PLDF 26DC5254801299

• • • • • • • • • • • •

Kale-Shallot Frittata

This recipe also works well with other greens such as spinach or chard.

Serves 4
Extra-virgin olive oil spray
1 large shallot
½–1 bunch kale, rinsed and thinly sliced (about 4 cups; leaves only)
1 Tablespoon extra-virgin olive oil
⅛ teaspoon sea salt
6 small, marinated, sun-dried (or roasted) tomatoes (packed in olive oil and herbs)
6 teaspoons goat cheese (optional)
2 Tablespoons shredded Parmesan cheese
8 medium eggs
½ cup whole milk
¼ teaspoon dried thyme (or 1 teaspoon fresh)
⅛ teaspoon pepper

Prepare a pie dish by coating it lightly with cooking spray. Preheat oven to 350°F.

In a large, nonstick skillet, sauté the shallot and kale in the olive oil over medium heat, until kale is wilted and shallots are aromatic. Sprinkle with sea salt and stir until well combined.

Place the kale mixture in the pie dish, covering the bottom evenly. Add the sundried tomatoes on top of the kale, evenly spaced in a circular pattern. Do the same with each teaspoon of goat cheese. Sprinkle the top with Parmesan cheese. Set aside.

In a separate bowl, whisk together the eggs, milk, thyme, and pepper. Then pour the mixture on top of kale mixture in the pie plate.

Carefully place the pie plate in the oven on the center rack. Bake for approximately 35 minutes, or until egg has set and the top is just starting to brown. Allow to cool at least 15 minutes before slicing. Delicious on it's own or served with a small side salad or whole-grain toast.

Per Serving: 250 Calories; 18g Fat (5g Sat.); 15g Protein; 6g Carbohydrate; 1g Dietary Fiber; 382mg Cholesterol; 313mg Sodium.

• • • • • • • • • • • •

Lentil and Sweet Potato Stew

Serves 8
4 cups low-sodium vegetable (or chicken) broth (or water), divided
1¼ cups lentils, rinsed
2 cups cooked sweet potatoes, peeled and cubed
½ onion, diced
½ cup diced celery
2 garlic cloves, minced
1 teaspoon tamari soy sauce
1 teaspoon cumin
½ teaspoon coriander
1½ cups diced zucchini

1½ cups chopped broccoli florets

In a large pot or Dutch oven, combine 3 cups vegetable broth with lentils; bring to a low boil. Reduce heat to medium and cook until lentils are barely tender (about 20 to 30 minutes).

Add sweet potatoes, onion, celery, garlic, additional 1 cup broth, tamari, cumin, and coriander. Cook uncovered on medium heat, stirring occasionally, for about 40 minutes.

Add zucchini and broccoli, and continue to heat another 10 minutes, until veggies are tender. Serve warm in shallow bowls. Makes eight 1-cup servings.

Per Serving: 399 Calories; 1g Fat (trace Sat.); 32g Protein; 69g Carbohydrate; 33g Dietary Fiber; 0mg Cholesterol; 135mg Sodium.

• • • • • • • • • • • •

Mango-Avocado Salsa

This salsa is loaded with vitamin C. Mangoes are also a great source of beta-carotene and fiber. Avocados provide heart-healthy mono-unsaturated fat as well as glutathione, which is a powerful anticancer antioxidant. And cilantro is a natural detoxifier.

Serves 4
1 avocado, peeled, pitted, and chopped
1 mango, peeled, pitted, and chopped
1 Tablespoon minced cilantro
1 cup halved cherry tomatoes
2 Tablespoons lime juice
½ teaspoon sea salt
1 jalapeño pepper, seeded and minced

Lightly toss all ingredients together in a medium, nonmetal bowl. Refrigerate until ready to serve. We typically serve this salsa on top of fish or with a side of chips or rice crackers.

Per Serving: 126 Calories; 8g Fat (1g Sat.); 2g Protein; 15g Carbohydrate; 3g Dietary Fiber; 0mg Cholesterol; 245mg Sodium.

• • • • • • • • • • • •

Mediterranean Lemon Chicken with Dill and Vegetable Rice

Serves 4
Chicken:
2 Tablespoons plain Greek yogurt
2 Tablespoons extra-virgin olive oil
1 lemon, zested and juiced (2 to 3 Tablespoons of juice)
1 Tablespoon red-wine vinegar
4 garlic cloves, minced or pressed
1 teaspoon paprika
1 Tablespoon dried oregano
1 teaspoon sea salt
¼ teaspoon pepper
2 boneless skinless chicken breasts (1 pound), pounded thin and halved
Cooking oil spray

Dill-and-vegetable rice:
2 cups low-sodium chicken or vegetable broth
3 Tablespoons extra-virgin olive oil, divided
1 cup uncooked brown rice

2 cups baby spinach, rinsed well and dry

½ red bell pepper, finely diced

½ cucumber, peeled, seeded, and finely diced

¼ small red onion, finely diced

6 ounces cherry tomatoes, halved (about 1 full cup)

¼ cup crumbled feta cheese (about 1 ounce; optional)

1 Tablespoon chopped dill

1 lemon, zested and juiced

½ teaspoon salt

¼ teaspoon black pepper

To make chicken:

Combine the Greek yogurt, olive oil, lemon zest and juice, vinegar, garlic, paprika, oregano, salt, and pepper in a small bowl to create a marinade. Pour marinade into a nonmetal bowl (preferably glass) or Ziploc bag and add chicken, making sure to coat completely. Marinate for at least an hour, overnight if possible. In a pinch, give it at least 20 minutes.

Note: the rice will take more than 35 minutes to prepare and cook, so you should get that started before you proceed with baking the chicken.

When ready to cook, preheat oven to 400°F and move the oven rack to the top third. Line a baking sheet or broiler pan with parchment paper or foil and coat with cooking oil spray.

Remove chicken from marinade and lay out evenly on the baking sheet. Place into the oven and bake for 12 to 15 minutes, or until the chicken is cooked through (no longer pink in the middle). Discard any leftover marinade.

To make dill and vegetable rice:

Pour the broth and 1 tablespoon of olive oil into a medium pot and bring to a low boil. Add rice, lower heat to simmer, and cover. Allow the rice to absorb the liquid, about 35 minutes.

Fluff the rice with a fork; cool slightly. If liquid evaporates before rice is fully cooked, add a bit of water, a few tablespoons at a time.

In a large bowl, combine the spinach, bell pepper, cucumber, onion, tomato, feta cheese, dill, lemon zest and juice, salt, pepper, and remaining 2 tablespoons olive oil; stir to combine. Set aside.

Once the rice is slightly cooled, add it to the large bowl of vegetables and stir to combine.

To serve, divide the warm rice on four separate plates, topping each with half a chicken breast, while still warm from the oven.

Per Serving: 536 Calories; 22g Fat (4g Sat.); 38g Protein; 48g Carbohydrate; 3g Dietary Fiber; 75mg Cholesterol; 1122mg Sodium.

• • • • • • • • • • • • •

Pacific Sole with Orange-Shallot Sauce

Look for Pacific sole (flounder), as Atlantic species are on the Monterey Bay Aquarium list of fish to avoid (due to overfishing).

Serves 4
⅓ cup almond meal/flour
½ teaspoon salt
Freshly ground pepper
1 pound Pacific flounder (sole or haddock fillets)
1 Tablespoon extra-virgin olive oil
1 large shallot, finely chopped (about ⅓ cup)
½ cup dry white wine
1 cup freshly squeezed orange juice (about 4 medium oranges)
2 heaping teaspoons Dijon mustard
2 teaspoons butter
2 Tablespoons chopped parsley

Mix the almond meal, salt, and pepper to taste in a shallow dish; thoroughly dredge fish fillets in the mixture. Set aside.

Heat oil in a large nonstick skillet over medium-high heat until shimmering but not smoking. Add the fish and cook until lightly browned and just opaque in the center, 3 to 4 minutes per side. (Do not overcook, as fish will continue to cook after it is removed from the heat.) Transfer to a plate and cover loosely with foil.

Place the shallot in the pan and cook over medium-high heat, stirring often, until softened and beginning to brown (about 3 minutes). Add the wine and bring to a simmer, scraping up any browned bits. Cook until most of the liquid has evaporated, 1 to 2 minutes. Add the orange juice and mustard; bring to a boil. Reduce heat to low and simmer until the sauce thickens a bit, about 5 minutes. Add the butter and parsley, and stir until the butter has melted.

Transfer fish to individual plates, top with sauce, and serve.

Per Serving: 222 Calories; 7g Fat; (2g Sat.); 23g Protein; 6g Carbohydrates; 0g Dietary Fiber; 59mg Cholesterol; 237mg Sodium.

•   •   •   •   •   •   •   •   •   •   •   •   •

Pork Tenderloin with Blueberry Sauce

Serves 4
Cooking oil spray
1 pound pork tenderloin (¾ to 1 pound)
½ teaspoon salt, divided
¼ teaspoon freshly ground black pepper, divided
1 Tablespoon extra-virgin olive oil
2 Tablespoons butter, divided
2 medium onions, sliced
2 Tablespoons sugar or honey

¼ cup port wine or sweet sherry
2 Tablespoons balsamic vinegar
1 cup fresh or frozen blueberries

Preheat oven to broil.

Spray a light coating of cooking oil on top of pork and sprinkle with ⅛ teaspoon each salt and pepper. Set aside.

Heat cast-iron skillet to medium high. Pour in the olive oil plus 1 tablespoon butter, then add pork and brown on all sides.

Transfer pork to a broiling pan and broil, turning occasionally, until cooked through (about 10 to 15 minutes). Remove to a platter and cover to keep warm.

In the same skillet used to brown the pork, melt the remaining 1 tablespoon of butter over medium heat. Add the onions, and remaining ⅜ teaspoon salt and ⅛ teaspoon pepper; cook until onions begin to wilt, about 10 minutes. Stir in sugar and continue cooking (and stirring) until onions are caramelized, about 3 more minutes. Add port, balsamic, and blueberries; bring to a boil, still stirring. Remove from heat.

Thinly slice the pork and serve with sauce.

Per Serving: 329 Calories; 11g Fat (5g Sat.); 20g Protein; 37g Carbohydrate; 6g Dietary Fiber; 51mg Cholesterol; 365mg Sodium.

•   •   •   •   •   •   •   •   •   •   •

Power Ranch Salad

Serves 2
Dressing:
1 small shallot, peeled
½ cup nonfat cottage cheese

2 Tablespoons reduced-fat mayonnaise
2 Tablespoons plain Greek yogurt
¼ cup lowfat buttermilk
2 Tablespoons white-wine vinegar
1 Tablespoon chopped dill
¼ teaspoon salt
¼ teaspoon freshly ground pepper

Salad:
6 cups mixed salad greens
1 cup shredded carrots
2 Tablespoons chopped red onion
10 cherry tomatoes
4 slices roast turkey breast (3 ounces), cut up
¼ cup dried organic cranberries or goji berries, to serve

To prepare dressing:
Combine the shallot, cottage cheese, mayonnaise, yogurt, buttermilk, and vinegar in a blender and process until smooth (about 1 minute), stopping to scrape down the sides as necessary. Add dill, salt, and pepper and process until combined. (Makes about 1¼ cups.)

To make salad and serve:
Toss greens, carrots, onion, and tomatoes with ¼ cup dressing in a large bowl until coated. Divide between 2 plates and arrange turkey on top of each. Sprinkle both with cranberries and serve. Makes two 4-cup servings.

Per Serving: 180 Calories; 4g Fat (1g Sat.); 21g Protein; 19g Carbohydrates; 6g Dietary Fiber; 27mg Cholesterol; 757mg Sodium.

• • • • • • • • • • • •

Quinoa and Black Bean Salad

Serves 5
1 Tablespoon extra-virgin olive oil
4 teaspoons lime juice
¼ teaspoon cumin
¼ teaspoon coriander
1 Tablespoon chopped cilantro
2 Tablespoons diced scallions
2 cups cooked quinoa (1 cup uncooked)
1½ cups (cooked or canned) black beans, rinsed and drained
2 cups diced tomatoes
1 cup diced red bell pepper
Salt and pepper

In a small bowl, whisk together the oil, lime juice, cumin, coriander, cilantro, and scallions; set aside.

Combine quinoa, beans, tomatoes, and bell peppers in a large bowl. Add dressing and toss well to combine thoroughly. Season lightly with salt and pepper as desired.

Serve cold or at room temperature.

Per Serving: 245 Calories; 5g Fat (1g Sat.); 10g Protein; 42g Carbohydrate; 8g Dietary Fiber; 0mg Cholesterol; 18mg Sodium.

. . . .

Roasted Beet Salad with Chicken, Goat Cheese, and Walnuts

Serves 4
1 head butter lettuce, rinsed well and gently dried
6 small beets, roasted, peeled, and sliced
½ red onion, sliced
16 ounces cooked chicken breast, cubed or sliced
4 Tablespoons extra-virgin olive oil
1 Tablespoon lemon juice
2 teaspoons dried dill
1 teaspoon Dijon mustard
Salt and pepper
2 ounces goat cheese, crumbled (about ¼ cup), to serve
2 Tablespoons chopped walnuts, to serve

Arrange butter lettuce on four dinner plates, and top each with equal portions of sliced beets, onion, and chicken. Set aside.

Whisk together olive oil, lemon juice, dill, and mustard in a small bowl. Add salt and pepper to taste.

To serve, drizzle dressing over each salad, and sprinkle with goat cheese and walnuts.

Per Serving: 457 Calories; 28g Fat (8g Sat.); 36g Protein; 16g Carbohydrate; 5g Dietary Fiber; 92mg Cholesterol; 230mg Sodium.

· · · · · · · · · · · ·

Stuffed Peppers

Serves 4

1 cup uncooked quinoa or short-grain brown rice
2 cups water or low-sodium chicken broth
4 medium red bell peppers (or variety of colored bell peppers)
1 Tablespoon extra-virgin olive oil
1 small onion, diced
1 garlic clove, minced
1 chicken (or tempeh) sausage link, chopped
½ cup chopped broccoli
¼ cup pine nuts
1 teaspoon ground cumin
½ small zucchini, diced
½ cup chopped spinach
1 Tablespoon chopped oregano
¼ teaspoon sea salt (optional)
2 ounces crumbled feta cheese (about ¼ cup)
Cooking oil spray

Combine quinoa with 2 cups of water or chicken broth in a medium-sized pot and bring to a boil. Lower the heat, cover, and simmer. Set your timer and check after 13 minutes, stirring or fluffing the quinoa with a fork before replacing the cover. Turn off heat and allow to sit.

While quinoa is cooking, slice the tops off the bell peppers about ½ inch down from the stem (don't throw away tops). Rinse the bell peppers, and remove the seeds and ribs.

Fill a large pot with water and heat until boiling. Once the water reaches boiling, submerge the (whole) bell peppers and allow them to simmer for about five minutes. Remove to a large colander and set aside to drain (or you can set them upside down on a paper towel or two). Note that the peppers can be prepared ahead of time and refrigerated until ready to assemble.

Chop the bell pepper tops that you set aside by cutting off any remaining bell pepper surrounding the stem (making sure it is well rinsed), then dice and add to a medium-sized bowl. Set aside.

Heat olive oil over medium-high heat in a large skillet. Add the onion, garlic, and sausage and stir-fry for about 5 minutes. Now add the reserved chopped bell pepper tops and broccoli, and cook another 5 minutes. Throw in the pine nuts and cumin, and stir for about a minute before adding the zucchini, spinach, oregano, and salt. Stir for another 3 minutes, then remove from the heat and stir in the quinoa and feta.

Preheat oven to 425°F. Set the bell peppers (cut side up) in a large rectangular baking dish that has been coated with cooking oil spray or lined with parchment paper. Fill each bell pepper with ¼ of the quinoa and veggie mixture. (If you have prepared the peppers ahead of time and they have been refrigerated, allow about 30 minutes for cooking.)

If you find you have extra quinoa-vegetable filling left over (meaning your peppers are overflowing), you can save it for another meal or heat it and serve it along side the peppers in a shallow bowl.

Per Serving: 290 Calories; 12g Fat (3g Sat.); 12g Protein; 36g Carbohydrate; 5g Dietary Fiber; 23mg Cholesterol; 340mg Sodium.

• • • • • • • • • • • • •

Stuffed Squash

Serves 4

2 medium-size winter squash (acorn or delicata work well)

Cooking oil spray

2 Tablespoons extra-virgin olive oil or melted butter, divided

½ cup chopped onion

½ cup chopped celery

2 cups chopped spinach

1 Tablespoon chopped sage

2 cups cooked wild or brown rice

½ cup dried cranberries

½ cup chopped pistachios

1 Tablespoon pure maple syrup or additional extra-virgin olive oil
    (optional)

Cut squash in half horizontally (not stem to stem) and remove seeds, scraping away any excess "stringiness." (If using delicata squash, just cut the squash in half and remove the seeds.)

Set squash in a large baking dish or roasting pan coated with cooking oil spray (cut side up) and coat the inside of each squash half with olive oil (about ¾ teaspoon per half).

Preheat oven to 375°F.

In a large skillet, heat 1½ tablespoons olive oil or butter over medium high heat. Add onion and celery, and sauté for about 5 minutes, stirring frequently. Add spinach and sage, and sauté another 3 minutes or so, until the spinach is fully wilted. Remove from heat.

In a large mixing bowl, combine the onion mixture and rice. Stir in cranberries and pistachios, and mix well.

Place ¼ of the mixture (about ¾ cup) in the cavity of each squash. Drizzle the tops with a bit of maple syrup (or you can drizzle the maple syrup inside of the squash prior to filling it). Alternatively, you can drizzle with a bit of olive oil.

Bake for about 40 minutes, or until squash is soft and top is lightly browned. Allow to cool a bit before serving (squash contents will be very hot).

Per Serving: 277 Calories; 12g Fat (2g Sat.); 9g Protein; 38g Carbohydrate; 6g Dietary Fiber; 0mg Cholesterol; 34mg Sodium.

· · · · · · · · · · · ·

Sweet Potato Turkey Tacos with Black Beans

Serves 4
2 Tablespoons extra-virgin olive oil, divided
1 medium yellow onion, chopped
1 medium sweet potato, peeled and cut into small cubes
1 teaspoon salt, plus more to taste
1 pound ground turkey breast or thigh
2 garlic cloves, minced
1 teaspoon dried oregano
2 teaspoons cumin
¼ cup tomato paste
2 teaspoons paprika
1 pinch cayenne pepper
½ teaspoon black pepper
8 corn tortillas (6-inch)
1 can (15-ounces) low-sodium black beans, rinsed and drained (to serve)

Garnishes:
½ head romaine lettuce, shredded
1 medium tomato, diced
½ cup Mexican-blend shredded cheese
4 Tablespoons plain Greek yogurt
1 Tablespoon fresh lime juice
2 Tablespoons chopped cilantro

Heat 1 tablespoon of the oil in a large, nonstick skillet over medium-high heat. Once hot, add the onion and sweet potato. Sprinkle with salt (to taste), lower heat to medium, and sauté until potatoes are soft and onion is translucent (5 to 7 minutes). Remove from heat and set aside.

In another large skillet, combine turkey, garlic, oregano, cumin, tomato paste, paprika, cayenne pepper, 1 teaspoon salt, and black pepper. Cook over medium heat until meat is browned and cooked through (7 to 10 minutes). Add sweet potato mixture and stir to incorporate. Remove from heat, cover, and set aside.

Warm tortillas on the stove over a low, open flame or wrap in a damp towel and microwave for 15 to 20 seconds.

Serve 2 tacos per person filled with ¼ cup of turkey–sweet potato mixture plus 2 tablespoons black beans. Garnish with a sprinkle of cheese, a dollop of Greek yogurt, and other desired garnishes as listed.

Per Serving: 551 Calories; 27g Fat (7g Sat.); 39g Protein; 45g Carbohydrate; 7g Dietary Fiber; 106mg Cholesterol; 1053mg Sodium.

•   •   •   •   •   •   •   •   •   •   •

Tuscan-Style Tuna Salad

Serves 4
2 cans (6-ounce) chunk light tuna, drained

1 can (15-ounce) small white beans (such as cannellini or great
   northern), rinsed and drained
10 cherry tomatoes, quartered
4 scallions, trimmed and sliced
2 Tablespoons extra-virgin olive oil
2 Tablespoons lemon juice
¼ teaspoon salt
Freshly ground pepper

Combine all ingredients in a medium bowl and toss gently to mix.
Refrigerate until ready to serve.

You can enjoy this salad atop a bed of greens, or in a small (6-inch)
whole grain pita, or on top of 2 brown rice cakes.

Per Serving: 253 Calories; 8g Fat (1g Sat.); 31g Protein; 20g Carbohydrates; 6g Dietary Fiber; 53mg Cholesterol; 453mg Sodium.

•   •   •   •   •   •   •   •   •   •   •

White Bean and Barley Soup

Serves 4
1 cup cannelini beans, soaked overnight*
2 Tablespoons extra-virgin olive oil
2 large stalks celery and leafy tops, chopped
1 medium onion, chopped
1 garlic clove, minced
4 cups low-sodium chicken or vegetable broth
4 cups water
½ cup uncooked barley (or short-grain brown rice), rinsed
2 medium carrots, chopped
½ teaspoon dried oregano

½ teaspoon dried thyme
1 can (28-ounce) tomatoes
2 cups chopped spinach
¼ cup chopped parsley
2 tablespoons red-wine vinegar
Salt and pepper

Soak beans overnight in water. Discard the water, rinse the beans, and set aside to drain.

In the meantime, heat the oil in a large saucepan. Add celery, onion, and garlic and sauté 2 to 3 minutes. Add the broth and water, then the beans, barley, carrots, oregano, and thyme. Simmer 1 to 1½ hours, or until beans are tender.

Stir in tomatoes, spinach, parsley, and vinegar, stirring well to combine. Continue to simmer on a low until spinach is wilted. Season with salt and pepper, and serve warm.

*For a super-quick version of this soup, you can use canned beans. Just reduce the water to 1 cup and the simmering time to 40 minutes.

Per Serving: 383 Calories; 8g Fat (1g Sat.); 18g Protein; 64g Carbohydrate; 6g Dietary Fiber; 0mg Cholesterol; 362mg Sodium.

NOTES

Introduction

1. World Health Organization, Media Centre, "Depression," Fact Sheet no. 369, World Health Organization (October 2012): http://www.who.int/mediacentre/factsheets/fs369/en/.
2. National Center for Health Statistics, "Health, United States, 2011: With Special Feature on Socioeconomic Status and Health," US Department of Health and Human Services, Hyattsville, MD, (May 2012): 42, http://www.cdc.gov/nchs/data/hus/hus11.pdf.
3. Susan Adams, "New Survey: Majority of Employees Dissatisfied." *Forbes.com* (May 18, 2012): http://www.forbes.com/sites/susanadams/2012/05/18/new-survey-majority-of-employees-dissatisfied/.
4. IMS Health, "Total Unaudited and Audited Global Pharmaceutical Market (2003–2012)," IMS Health Market Prognosis (June 2013): 1, http://www.imshealth.com/deployedfiles/imshealth/Global/Content/Corporate/Press%20Room/Total_World_Pharma_Market_Topline_metrics_2012.pdf.

NOTES

Part I: THINK
Chapter 1

1. Jody Stevenson, "From Crazy Busy to Balance and Bliss," presented at Tea Talks for Women, October 13, 2013, Mile Hi Church, Lakewood, CO.
2. Julianne Holt-Lunstad, Timothy B. Smith, and J. Bradley Layton, "Social Relationships and Mortality Risk: A Meta-analytic Review," *PLoS Med* 7, no. 7 (2010): e1000316. doi:10.1371/journal.pmed.1000316.
3. N. Waxler-Morrison, T.G. Hislop, B. Mears, and L. Kan, "Effects of Social Relationships on Survival for Women with Breast Cancer: A Prospective Study." *Social Science & Medicine* 33, no. 2 (1991): 177–183.
4. His Holiness the 14th Dalai Lama, "His Holiness the Dalai Lama's Vision for a Future Free Tibet," The Pictorial Portrait Project, February 26, 1992, http://www.dalailama -archives.org/texts.php?pageID=9.

Chapter 2

1. Nicole Martins and Kristen Harrison, "Racial and Gender Differences in the Relationship Between Children's Television Use and Self-Esteem: A Longitudinal Panel Study," *Communication Research* 39, no. 3 (2011): 338.
2. Barbara J. Wilson, "Media and Children's Aggression, Fear, and Altruism," *The Future of Children* 18, no. 1 (Spring 2008): 87–118. http://futureofchildren.org/futureof children/publications/docs/18_01_05.pdf.
3. Yonas E. Geda, Lon S. Schneider, Laura N. Gitlin, David S. Miller, Gwenn S. Smith, Joanne Bell, Jovier Evans, Michael Lee, Anton Porsteinsson, Krista L. Lanctôt, Paul B. Rosenberg, David L. Sultzer, Paul T. Francis, Henry Brodaty, Prasad P. Padala, Chiadikaobi U. Onyike, Luis Agüera Ortiz, Sonia Ancoli-Israel, Donald L. Bliwise, Jennifer L. Martin, Michael V. Vitiello, Kristine Yaffe, Phyllis Zee, Nathan Herrmann, Robert A. Sweet, Clive Ballard, Ni A. Khin, Cara Alfaro, Patrick S. Murray, Susan Schultz, and Constantine G. Lyketsos, "Neuropsychiatric Symptoms in Alzheimer's Disease: Past Progress and Anticipation of the Future," *Alzheimer's & Dementia* 9, no. 5 (2013): 602–608.
4. Ai Ikeda, Joel Schwartz, Junenette L. Peters, Shona Fang, Avron Spiro III, David Sparrow, Pantel Vokonas, and Laura D. Kubzansky, "Optimism in Relation to Inflammation and Endothelial Dysfunction in Older Men: the VA Normative Aging Study," *Psychosomatic Medicine* 73, no. 8 (2011): 664–671.

Chapter 3

1. Jon Kabat-Zinn, "Jon Kabat-Zinn Defines Mindfulness." NourFoundation, YouTube (February, 23, 2013): http://www.youtube.com/watch?v=wPNEmxWSNxg.

2. J. David Creswell, Michael R. Irwin, Lisa J. Burklund, Matthew D. Lieberman, Jesusa M. Arevalo, Jeffrey Ma, Elizabeth Crab Breen, and Steven W. Cole, "Mindfulness-Based Stress Reduction Training Reduces Loneliness and Pro-inflammatory Gene Expression in Older Adults: A Small Randomized Controlled Trial," *Brain Behavior and Immunity* 26, no. 7 (2012): 1095–1101.

3. Matthijs Kox, Monique Stoffels, Sanne P. Smeekens, Nens van Alfen, Marc Gomes, Thijs M.H. Eijsvogels, Maria T.E. Hopman, Johannes G. van der Hoeven, Mihai G. Netea, and Peter Pickkers, "The Influence of Concentration/Meditation on Autonomic Nervous System Activity and the Innate Immune Response: A Case Study," *Psychosomatic Medicine* 74, no. 5 (2012): 489–494.

4. Madhav Goyal, Sonal Singh, Erica M.S. Sibinga, Neda F. Gould, Anastasia Rowland-Seymour, Ritu Sharma, Zackary Berger, Dana Sleicher, David D. Maron, Hasan M. Shihab, Padmini D. Ranasinghe, Shauna Linn, Shonali Saha, Eric E. Bass, and Jennifer A. Haythornthwaite, "Meditation Programs for Psychological Stress and Well-being: A Systematic Review and Meta-analysis." *Journal of the American Medical Association* 174, no. 3 (January 6, 2014): 357–368.

5. Bonnie Tarantino, Michael Earley, Donna Audia, Christopher D'Adamo, and Brian Berman, "Qualitative and Quantitative Evaluation of a Pilot Integrative Coping and Resiliency Program for Healthcare Professionals," *Explore* (NY) 9, no. 1 (January–February 2013): 44–47.

6. Victoria Tilney McDonough, "The Role of Mindfulness, Meditation, and Prayer After Brain Injury," Brainline.org (Accessed March 7, 2014): www.brainline.org /content/2009/12/the-role-of-mindfulness-meditation-and-prayer-after-brain -injury.html.

7. Elizabeth A. Hoge, Eric Bui, Luana Marques, Christina A. Metcalf, Laura K. Morris, Donald J. Robinaugh, John J. Worthington, Mark H. Pollack, and Naomi M. Simon, "Randomized Controlled Trial of Mindfulness Meditation for Generalized Anxiety Disorder: Effects on Anxiety and Stress Reactivity," *Journal of Clinical Psychiatry* 74, no. 8 (2013): 786–792.

Chapter 4

1. Ruut Veenhoven, "Healthy Happiness: Effects of Happiness on Physical Health and the Consequences for Preventive Health Care," *Journal of Happiness Studies* 9, no. 3 (2008): 449.

2. Martin Seligman, *Authentic Happiness: Using the New Positive Psychology to Realize Your Potential for Lasting Fulfillment* (New York: Free Press, 2002), 134.

3. B.L. Smith, "Inappropriate Prescribing," *American Psychological Association* 43, no. 6 (2012): 36.

4. Karma Ura, Sabina Alkire, Tshoki Zangmo, and Karma Wangdi, "A Short Guide To Gross National Happiness Index," The Centre for Bhutan Studies (2012): 6–10,

http://www.grossnationalhappiness.com/wp-content/uploads/2012/04/Short-GNH
-Index-edited.pdf.

5. M. de Vanna and R. Rigamonti, "Oral S-adenosyl-l-methionine in Depression," *Current Therapeutic Research* 52, no. 3 (1992): 478–485.

6. Consuelo H. Wilkins, Stanley J. Birge, Yvette I. Sheline, and John C. Morris, "Vitamin D Deficiency is Associated with Low Mood and Worse Cognitive Performance in Older Adults," *American Journal of Geriatric Psychiatry* 14, no. 12 (2006): 1032–1040.

7. Lee S. Berk, Stanley A. Tan, William F. Fry, Barbara J. Napier, Jerry W. Lee, Richard W. Hubbard, John E. Lewis, and William C. Eby, "Neuroendocrine and Stress Hormone Changes During Mirthful Laughter," *American Journal of the Medical Sciences* 298, no. 6 (1989): 390–396.

8. Ibid.

9. Ibid.

10. Eun A. Cho and Hyun Ei Oh, "Effects of Laughter Therapy on Depression, Quality of Life, Resilience and Immune Responses in Breast Cancer Survivors," *Journal of Korean Academy of Nursing* 41, no. 3 (2011): 285–293.

11. Mary P. Bennett, Janice M. Zeller, Lisa Rosenberg, and Judith McCann, "The Effect of Mirthful Laughter on Stress and Natural Killer Cell Activity," *Alternative Therapies in Health and Medicine* 9, no. 2 (2003): 38–45.

12. R. I. M. Dunbar, Rebecca Baron, Anna Frangou, Eiluned Pearce, Edwin J. C. van Leeuwen, Julie Stow, Giselle Partridge, Ian MacDonald, Vincent Barra, and Mark van Vugt, "Social Laughter is Correlated with an Elevated Pain Threshold," *Proceedings of the Royal Society B: Biological Sciences* 279, no. 1731 (2012): 1161–1167.

13. James H. Fowler and Nicholas A. Christakis, "Dynamic Spread of Happiness in a Large Social Network: Longitudinal Analysis Over 20 Years in the Framingham Heart Study," *British Medical Journal* 337, no. a 2338 (2008): 1–9.

14. John F. Helliwell, Richard Layard, and Jeffrey D. Sachs, et al., "World Happiness Report 2013." The Earth Institute, Columbia University (New York: UN Sustainable Development Solutions Network) Accessed March 8, 2014: http://issuu.com/earth institute/docs/worldhappinessreport2013_online.

15. Robert A. Emmons and Michael E. McCullough, "Counting Blessings Versus Burdens: Experimental Studies of Gratitude and Subjective Well-being in Daily Life," *Journal of Personality and Social Psychology* 84, no. 2 (2003): 377–389.

16. Michael E. McCullough, Joanne A. Tsang, and Robert A. Emmons, "Gratitude in Intermediate Affective Terrain: Links of Grateful Moods to Individual Differences and Daily Emotional Experience," *Journal of Personality and Social Psychology* 86, no. 2 (2004): 295–309.

17. Robert Emmons, *Thanks!: How Practicing Gratitude Can Make You Happier* (New York: Houghton Mifflin, 2008), 201.

18. Tali Sharot, Alison M. Riccardi, Candace M. Raio, and Elizabeth A. Phelps, "Neural Mechanisms Mediating Optimism Bias," *Nature* 1, no. 450 (2007): 102–105.
19. Miriam A. Mosing, Sarah E. Medland, Allan McRae, Joseph George Landers, Margaret J. Wright, Nicholas G. Martin, "Genetic Influences on Life Span and its Relationship to Personality: A 16-year Follow-up Study of a Sample of Aging Twins," *Psychosomatic Medicine* 74, no. 1 (2012): 16–22.
20. Jeff C. Huffman, Carol A. Mastromauro, Julia K. Boehm, Rita Seabrook, Gregory L. Fricchione, John W. Denninger, and Sonja Lyubomirsky, "Development of a Positive Psychology Intervention for Patients with Acute Cardiovascular Disease," *Heart International* 6, no. 2 (2011): e14.
21. Jeffrey J. Froh, Todd B. Kashdan, Kathleen M. Ozimkowski, and Norman Miller, "Who Benefits the Most from a Gratitude Intervention in Children and Adolescents?: Examining Positive Affect as a Moderator," *The Journal of Positive Psychology* 4, no. 5 (2009): 408–422.
22. Rollin McCraty, Bob Barrios-Choplin, Deborah Rozman, Mike Atkinson, and Alan D. Watkins, "The Impact of a new Emotional Self-Management Program on Stress, Emotions, Heart Rate Variability, Dhea and Cortisol," *Integrative Physiological and Behavioral Science* 32, no. 2 (1998): 151–170.

Part Two: EAT

1. Emily K. Anderson, Dario A. Gutierrez, Arion Kennedy, and Alyssa H. Hasty, "Weight Cycling Increases T-Cell Accumulation in Adipose Tissue and Impairs Systemic Glucose Tolerance," *Diabetes* 62, no. 9 (2013): 3180–3188.

Chapter 5

1. Joshua Rosenthal, *Integrative Nutrition* (New York: Integrative Nutrition Publishing, 2008), 142.

Chapter 6

1. Dario Giugliano, Antonio Ceriello, and Katherine Esposito, "The Effects of Diet on Inflammation: Emphasis on the Metabolic Syndrome," *Journal of the American College of Cardiology* 48, no. 4 (2006): 677–685.
2. Cynthia L. Ogden, Margaret D. Carroll, Brian K. Kit, and Katherine M. Flegal, "Prevalence of Obesity Among Adults: United States, 2011–2012," NCHS Data Brief no. 131 (October 2013): 1–2, http://www.cdc.gov/nchs/data/databriefs/db131.pdf.
3. Centers for Disease Control and Prevention, "National Diabetes Fact Sheet: National Estimates and General Information on Diabetes and Prediabetes in the United

States," U.S. Department of Health and Human Services, Centers for Disease Control and Prevention (2011): 1, http://www.cdc.gov/diabetes/pubs/pdf/ndfs_2011.pdf.

4. Centers for Disease Control and Prevention, "Prevalence of Doctor-Diagnosed Arthritis and Arthritis-Attributable Activity Limitation—United States, 2007–2009," *Morbidity and Mortality Weekly Report* 59, no. 39 (October 8, 2010): 1261–1265. http://www.cdc.gov/mmwr/pdf/wk/mm5939.pdf.

5. Liesi E. Hebert, Paul E. Scherr, J.L. Bienias, D. A. Bennett, and Denis A. Evans, "Alzheimer Disease in the US Population: Prevalence Estimates Using the 2000 Census," *Archives of Neurology* 60, no. 8 (2003): 1119–1122.

6. Catalina Alarcón de la Lastra and Isabel Villegas, "Resveratrol as an Anti-inflammatory and Anti-aging Agent: Mechanisms and Clinical Implications." *Molecular Nutrition & Food Research* 49, no. 5 (2005): 405–430.

7. Chibuike C. Udenigwe, Vanu R. Ramprasath, Rotimi E. Aluko, and Peter J.H. Jones, "Potential of Resveratrol in Anticancer and Anti-inflammatory Therapy," *Nutrition Review* 66, no. 8 (2008): 445–454.

8. J.E. Chavarro, T. L. Toth, S.M. Sadio, and R. Hauser, "Soy Food and Isoflavone Intake in Relation to Semen Quality Parameters Among Men from an Infertility Clinic," *Human Reproduction* 23, no. 11 (2008): 2584-2590; J. Seppen, "A diet containing the soy phytoestrogen genistein causes infertility in female rats partially deficient in UDP glucuronyltransferase," *Toxicology and Applied Pharmacology* 264, no. 3 (September 20, 2012): 335-342.

9. R.L. Divi, H.C. Chang, and D.R. Doerge, "Anti-thyroid Isoflavones from Soybean: Isolation, Characterization, and Mechanisms of Action," *Biochemical Pharmacology* 54, no. 10 (1997): 1087-1096.

10. D. Roccisano, M. Henneberg, and A. Saniotis, "A Possible Cause of Alzheimer's Dementia—Industrial Soy Foods," *Medical Hypotheses* 82, no. 3 (2014): 250-254.

11. C.R. D'Adamo and A. Sahin, "Soy Foods and Supplementation: A Review of Commonly Perceived Health Benefits and Risks," *Alternative Therapies in Health and Medicine* 20, Suppl 1 (2014): 39-51.

12. An Pan, Qi Sun, Adam M. Bernstein, Matthias B. Schulze, JoAnn E. Manson, Meir J. Stampfer, Walter C. Willett, and Frank B. Hu, "Red Meat Consumption and Mortality: Results From 2 Prospective Cohort Studies" *Archives of Internal Medicine* 172, no. 7 (2012): 555–563.

13. Ibid.

14. Anita W. Jones, *Healthy, Wealthy, and Wise: A Thorough and Balanced Analysis of Biblical Diet and Wellness from Genesis to Revelation* (Maitland, FL: Xulon Press, 2008), 137.

Chapter 7

1. Lisa R. Young and Marion Nestle, "Expanding Portion Sizes in the US Marketplace: Implications for Nutrition Counseling," *Journal of the American Dietetic Association*, 103 (2003): 231–234.
2. The North American Association for the Study of Obesity, "National Nutrition Summit Position Paper," Obesity Society (accessed November 18, 2013): http://www .obesity.org/publications/national-nutrition-summit-position-paper.htm.
3. Rick Unger, "Obesity Now Costs Americans More In HealthCare Spending Than Smoking," *Forbes Magazine* (last modified April 30, 2012): http://www.forbes.com /sites/rickungar/2012/04/30/obesity-now-costs-americans-more-in-healthcare -costs-than-smoking/.
4. Weight Control & Diabetes Research Center, "NWCR Facts," The National Weight Control Registry, Brown Medical School/The Miriam Hospital (accessed March 7, 2014): http://www.nwcr.ws/Research/.
5. Artemis Dona and Ioannis S. Arvanitoyannis, "Health Risks of Genetically Modified Foods," *Critical Reviews in Food Science and Nutrition* 49, no. 2 (2009): 164–175.
6. Paul Pestano, Etan Yeshua, and Jane Houlihan, "Sugar in Children's Cereals: Popular Brands Pack More Sugar Than Snack Cakes and Cookies," Environmental Working Group (December 2011): 4, http://static.ewg.org/reports/2011/cereals/pdf/2011 -EWG-Cereals-Report.pdf.
7. Yunsheng Ma, Jennifer A. Griffith, Lisa Chasan-Taber, Barbara C. Olendzki, Elizabeth Jackson, Edward J. Stanek III, Wenjun Li, Sherry L. Pagoto, Andrea R. Hafner, and Ira S. Ockene, "Association Between Dietary Fiber and Serum C-reactive Protein 1-3," *American Journal of Clinical Nutrition* 83, no. 4 (2006): 760–766.
8. Alicja Wolk, JoAnn E. Manson, Meir J. Stampfer, Graham A. Colditz, Frank B. Hu, Frank E. Speizer, Charles H. Hennekens, and Walter C. Willett, "Long-term Intake of Dietary Fiber and Decreased Risk of Coronary Heart Disease Among Women," *Journal of the American Medical Association* 281, no. 21 (1999): 1998–2004.
9. Frank B. Hu, "Plant-based Foods and Prevention of Cardiovascular Disease: an Overview," *American Journal of Clinical Nutrition*, 78, no. 3 (2003): 544S–551S.
10. Diane E. Threapleton, Darren C. Greenwood, Charlotte E. Evans, Christine L. Cleghorn, Camilla Nykjaer, Charlotte Woodhead, Janet E. Cade, Christopher P. Gale, and Victoria J. Burley, "Dietary Fibre Intake and Risk of Cardiovascular Disease: Systematic Review and Meta-analysis," *British Medical Journal* 19, no. 347 (2013): f6879

Chapter 8

1. R. Molteni, R.J. Barnard, Z. Ying, C.K. Roberts, and F. Gómez-Pinilla, "A High-fat, Refined Sugar Diet Reduces Hippocampal Brain-Derived Neurotropic Factor, Neuronal Plasticity, and Learning," *Neuroscience*, 112, no. 4 (2002): 803–814.

2. Norman B. Anderson, Katherine C. Nordal, Steven J. Breckler, David Ballard, Lynn Bufka, Luana Bossolo, Sophie Bethune, Angel Brownawell, Kate Kelly, "Stress in America Findings." American Psychological Association (November 9, 2010): 15, http://www.apa.org/news/press/releases/stress/2010/national-report.pdf.
3. Alexander Panossian, Georg Wikman, and J. Sarris, "Rosenroot (Rhodiola rosea): Traditional Use, Chemical Composition, Pharmacology and Clinical Efficacy," *Phytomedicine*, 17, no. 7 (2010): 481–493.
4. Reem Malouf and John Grimley Evans, "Folic Acid With or Without Vitamin B12 for the Prevention and Treatment of Healthy Elderly and Demented People," *The Cochrane Database of Systematic Reviews* 8, no. 4 (2008): CD004514.
5. Martha Clare Morris, Denis A. Evans, Julia L. Bienias, Christine C. Tangney, David A. Bennett, Robert S. Wilson, Neelum Aggarwal, and Julie Schneider, "Consumption of Fish and N-3 Fatty Acids and Risk of Incident Alzheimer Disease," *Archives of Neurology*, 60, no. 7 (2003): 940–946.
6. Shinichi Kuriyama, Atsushi Hozawa, Kaori Ohmori, Taichi Shimazu, Toshifumi Matsui, Satoru Ebihara, Shuichi Awata, Ryoichi Nagatomi, Hiroyuki Arai, and Ichiro Tsuji, "Green Tea Consumption and Cognitive Function: A Cross-Sectional Study from the Tsurugaya Project," *American Journal of Clinical Nutrition*, 83, no. 2 (2006): 355–361.

Part Three: MOVE

1. Centers for Disease Control and Prevention, "Facts About Physical Activity" (last modified February 5, 2014): http://www.cdc.gov/physicalactivity/data/facts.html.
2. Ali H. Mokdad, James S. Marks, Donna F. Stroup, Julie L. Gerberding, "Actual Causes of Death in the United States, 2000," *Journal of the American Medical Association*, 291, no. 10 (2004): 1238-1245.
3. Mark Hamer, Kim L. Lavoie, and Simon L. Bacon, "Taking up Physical Activity in Later Life and Healthy Ageing: the English Longitudinal Study of Ageing," *British Journal of Sports Medicine*, 48, no. 3 (2014): 239–243.
4. Ann Smith Barnes and Stephanie A. Coulter (ed.), "Obesity and Sedentary Lifestyles: Risk for Cardiovascular Disease in Women," *Texas Heart Institute Journal*, 39, no. 2 (2012): 224–227; Tatiana Y. Warren, Vaughn Barry, Steven P. Hooker, Xuemei Sui, Timothy S. Church, and Steven N. Blair, "Sedentary Behaviors Increase Risk of Cardiovascular Disease Mortality in Men," *Medicine and Science in Sports and Exercise*, 42, no. 5 (2010): 879–885.
5. J. Meikle, A. Al-Sarraf, M. Li, K. Grierson, and J. Frohlich, "Exercise in a Healthy Heart Program: A Cohort Study," *Clinical Medical Insights. Cardiology*, 15, no. 7 (2013): 145–151.

NOTES

Chapter 9

1. John Percy, "London 2012 Olympics: Brazil's Women Footballers Labelled Too Fat to Win Gold at Games by Defeated Coach," *The Telegraph* online (July 26, 2012): http://www.telegraph.co.uk/sport/olympics/football/9430979/London-2012-Olympics-Brazils-women-footballers-labelled-too-fat-to-win-gold-at-Games-by-defeated-coach.html.
2. Cheryl D. Fryar, Quiping Gu, Cynthia L. Ogden, "Anthropometric Reference Data for Children and Adults: United States, 2007–2010." National Center for Health Statistics, *Vital Health Statistics*, 11, no. 252 (2012): tables 4, 6, 10, 12, 19, 20. http://www.cdc.gov/nchs/data/series/sr_11/sr11_252.pdf.
3. Data from the National Health Survey, "Weight, Height, and Selected Body Dimensions Of Adults: United States—1960–1962," DHEW Publication No. (HRA), series 11, no. 8, 76-1074, U.S. Department of Health, Education, and Welfare, Public Health Service (Health Resources Administration, National Center for Health Statistics, Rockville, Maryland): 6–7, http://www.cdc.gov/nchs/data/series/sr_11/sr11_008.pdf.
4. Cynthia L. Ogden, Margaret D. Carroll, Brian K. Kit, and Katherine M. Flegal, "Prevalence of Obesity Among Adults: United States, 2011–2012," NCHS Data Brief, no. 131, National Center for Health Statistics, Center for Disease Control and Prevention, (last modified October 17, 2013): http://www.cdc.gov/nchs/data/databriefs/db131.htm.

Chapter 10

1. Timothy J. Schoenfeld, Pedro Rada, Pedro R. Pieruzzini, Brian Hsueh, and Elizabeth Gould, "Physical Exercise Prevents Stress-induced Activation of Granule Neurons and Enhances Local Inhibitory Mechanisms in the Dentate Gyrus. Exercise and Anxiety," *Journal of Neuroscience*, 33, no. 18 (2013): 7770–7777.
2. Karen M. Mustian, Lisa K. Sprod, Michelle Janelsins, Luke J. Peppone, and Supriya Mohile, "Exercise Recommendations for Cancer-Related Fatigue, Cognitive Impairment, Sleep Problems, Depression, Pain, Anxiety, and Physical Dysfunction: A Review," *Oncology & Hematology Review*, 8, no. 2 (2012): 81–88.
3. Michelle D. Holmes, Wendy Y. Chen, Diane Feskanich, Candyce H. Kroenke, and Graham A. Colditz, "Physical Activity and Survival After Breast Cancer Diagnosis," *Journal of the American Medical Association*, 293, no. 20 (2005): 2479–2486.
4. Hajo Adam and Adam D. Galinsky, "Enclothed Cognition," *Journal of Experimental Social Psychology*, 48, no. 4 (2012): 918–925.
5. Dan Buettner, *The Blue Zones: Lessons for Living Longer from the People Who've Lived the Longest* (Washington DC: The National Geographic Society, 2008), 4–5.

NOTES

Chapter 11

1. Hau Liu, Dena M. Bravata, Ingram Olkin, Smita Nayak, Brian Roberts, Alan M. Garber, and Andrew R. Hoffman, "Systematic Review: The Safety and Efficacy of Growth Hormone in the Healthy Elderly," *Annals of Internal Medicine* 146, no. 2 (2007): 104–115.
2. US Food and Drug Administration, "Import Alert 66-71," US Department of Health and Human Services: http://www.accessdata.fda.gov/cms_ia/importalert_204.html.
3. Richard J. Godfrey, Zahra Madgwick, and Gregory P. Whyte, "The Exercise-induced Growth Hormone Response in Athletes," *Sports Medicine* 33, no. 8 (2003): 599–613.
4. Mark D. Peterson, Ananda Sen, and Paul M. Gordon, "Influence of Resistance Exercise on Lean Body Mass in Aging Adults: a Meta-analysis," *Medicine and Science in Sports and Exercise*, 43, no. 2 (2011): 249–258.
5. Toshihiko Tsutsumi, Brian M. Don, Leonard D. Zaichkowsky, and Laura L. Delizonna, "Physical fitness and Psychological Benefits of Strength Training in Community Dwelling Older Adults," *Applied Human Science*, 16, no. 6 (1997): 257–266.
6. Sarita Kanojia, Vivek Kumar Sharma, Asha Gandhi, Raj Kapoor, Ajay Kukreja, and Senthil Kumar Subramanian, "Effect of Yoga on Autonomic Functions and Psychological Status During Both Phases of Menstrual Cycle in Young Healthy Females," *Journal of Clinical and Diagnostic Research* 7, no. 10 (2013): 2133–2139.

Chapter 12

1. Megumi Ida, Itsurou Ida, Naoki Wada, Makoto Sohmiya, Masayuki Tazawa, and Kenji Shirakura, "A Clinical Study of the Efficacy of a Single Session of Individual Exercise for Depressive Patients, Assessed by the Change in Saliva Free Cortisol Level," *Biopsychosocial Medicine* 7, no. 1 (2013): 18.
2. Jen Uscher and Jennifer Carr, "Physical Exercise Beefs Up the Brain." BrainFacts.org, (August 28 2013): http://www.brainfacts.org/across-the-lifespan/diet-and-exercise/articles/2013/physical-exercise-beefs-up-the-brain/.
3. Karen S. Krabbe, Erik L. Mortensen, Kirsten Avlund, Agnes N. Pedersen, Bente K. Pedersen, Torben Jørgensen, and Helle Bruunsgaard, "Brain-derived Neurotrophic Factor Predicts Mortality Risk in Older Women," *Journal of the American Geriatric Society* 57, no. 8 (2009): 1447–1452.
4. Dawn Podulka Coe, James M. Pivarnik, Christopher J. Womack, Mathew J. Reeves, and Robert M. Malina, "Health-related Fitness and Academic Achievement in Middle School Students," *Journal of Sports Medicine and Physical Fitness* 52, no. 6 (2012): 654–660.
5. Dawn Podulka Coe, James M. Pivarnik, Christopher J. Womack, Mathew J. Reeves, and Robert M. Malina, "Effect of Physical Education and Activity Levels on Aca-

demic Achievement in Children," *Medicine and Science in Sports and Exercise* 38, no. 8 (2006): 1515–1519.

6. William Thies and Laura Bleiler, "2013 Alzheimer's Disease Facts and Figures," *Alzheimer's and Dementia* 9, no 2 (Alzheimer's Association, 2013): 208–245.

7. Aron S. Buchman, P.A. Boyle, L. Yu, R.C. Shah, R.S. Wilson, and D.A. Bennett, "Total Daily Physical Activity and the Risk of AD and Cognitive Decline in Older Adults," *Neurology* 78, no. 17 (2012): 1323–1329.

8. Ibid.

9. Miia Kivipelto and Alina Solomon, "Alzheimer's Disease—The Ways of Prevention." *Journal of Nutrition, Health & Aging* 12, no. 1 (2008): 89S–94S.

10. Eric B. Larson, Li Wang, James D. Bowen, Wayne C. McCormick, Linda Teri, Paul Crane, and Walter Kukull, "Exercise is Associated with Reduced Risk for Incident Dementia Among Persons 65 Years of Age and Older," *Annals of Internal Medicine* 144, no. 2 (2006): 73–81.

11. Kirk I. Erickson, Andrea M. Weinsteina, and Oscar L. Lopez, "Physical Activity, Brain Plasticity, and Alzheimer's Disease," *Archives of Medical Research* 43, no. 8 (2012): 615–621.

12. Philip P. Foster, Kevin P. Rosenblatt, and Rodrigo O. Kuljiš, "Exercise-induced Cognitive Plasticity, Implications for Mild Cognitive Impairment and Alzheimer's Disease," *Frontiers in Neurology* 6, no. 2 (2011): 28.

Glossary

1. "Soybeans," Crops, GMO Compass (last modified December 3, 2008): http://www .gmocompass.org/eng/grocery_shopping/crops/19.genetically_modified_soybean .html. Accessed March 7, 2014.

2. National Research Council, "Dietary Reference Intakes: for Energy, Carbohydrate, Fiber, Fat, Fatty Acids, Cholesterol, Protein, and Amino Acids (Macronutrients)" (Washington D.C.: The National Academies Press, 2005): 339. http://www.nap.edu /catalog.php?record_id=10490.

3. "GMO Facts: Frequently Asked Questions," Non GMO Project (accessed January 30, 2014): http://www.nongmoproject.org/learn-more/.

GLOSSARY

Agave or Agave Nectar (or syrup) is a sweet substance, similar in taste and texture to honey but just a little sweeter, with a thinner consistency. Agave nectar is made up primarily of glucose and fructose and is considered a lower glycemic sweetener. It is a great honey substitute for vegans, but due to the high-fructose content, it may not be good for those with metabolic syndrome or diabetes.

Amaranth is a gluten-free seed grain grown around the world, primarily in Asia and North and South America. Amaranth is high in complete protein, especially the amino acid lysine. Nutty in flavor, it is great cooked up as a breakfast cereal or side dish, and the flour makes a great addition to any gluten-free baking mix. Use amaranth as a substitute for quinoa or brown rice.

Antioxidants are chemical substances that protect the body from the adverse effects of unstable oxygen molecules. While it is true that oxygen is an essential energy source for our cells, unstable oxygen can actually be toxic and damaging to our bodies. Unstable oxygen is what we have in free radicals. Free radicals are formed as a result of factors like excess exposure to the sun, cigarette smoke and air pollution, excess alcohol, and exposure to radiation. Free radicals can damage the body's cells and DNA, and interrupt the normal ability to reproduce healthy cells. Anti-oxidants fight back against free radical damage, which is why they are an essential part of TEMT. We can find antioxidants within the body, or we can find them in the foods we eat or the supplements we take. Green tea is one example of a beverage that contains naturally occurring antioxidants.

Cognitive Function is the ability to problem solve and process thoughts, and is related to intelligence, memory, speech, and comprehension.

Curry is best classified as a variety of spices that often includes curry leaves, turmeric, coriander, cumin, and red pepper—but the combination of spices can vary considerably, depending on the type of cuisine. Curry powder is available commercially, as is curry paste. The bright yellow color of curry powder is due to turmeric, which is known as a powerful anti-inflammatory agent.

Edamame are soybeans, still in their pods. They are usually boiled or steamed before eating and sprinkled lightly with sea salt. Edamame is found in most grocery stores and Asian markets in the frozen food section. It may also be found near the prepared food section, especially if the grocer offers sushi. We always recommend choosing organic when it comes to soy products since soy is one of the most popular genetically modified (GM) crops. (More than half of the world's soy crop is GM, and in the United States, about 85 percent of the soybean crops are GM soybeans.[1])

Essential Fatty Acids (EFAs) are necessary fats that humans cannot synthesize and must be obtained through diet. EFAs are long-chain polyunsaturated fatty acids derived from linolenic (ALA) (omega-3), linoleic (LA) (omega-6), and oleic acids. Both omega-3s and omega-6s decrease inflammation in the body and prevent certain chronic diseases. When balanced in the body, EFAs support the cardiovascular, reproductive, immune, and nervous systems. The Standard American Diet (SAD) is typically much higher in omega-6s compared to omega-3s, which can increase the risk for inflammation in the body. Too much omega-6 can actually promote inflammation. Eicosapentaenoic acid (EPA) and docosahexaenoic acid (DHA), the omega-3 fatty acids found in the fat of deep-sea, cold-water fish, have been shown to decrease inflammation and help prevent many chronic diseases. Flaxseed oil contains both omega-3 and omega-6 fatty acids—however the process of converting ALA from flaxseed oil into EPA and DHA is not always efficient; such is the case with most plant-based sources of omega-3s.

Research isn't clear at this point how well EFAs are converted to EPA and DHA, and it tends to vary considerably between individuals. Still, it is important for vegetarians to consume foods that are high in omega-3s since vegetarians typically consume high levels of omega-6s. Higher dietary omega-3 intakes are associated with decreased risk of cardiovascular disease and stroke. Best sources of omega-3s include wild salmon, walnuts, sardines, organic soybeans, shrimp, Brussels sprouts, hempseed, Brazil nuts, pumpkin seeds, mackerel, anchovies, cauliflower, winter squash, flaxseed, tuna, and avocado. Omega-6 sources include meat, poultry, eggs, nuts, seeds, most vegetable oils, coconut, and durum wheat.

Fiber is a type of carbohydrate that moves through the digestive tract basically unchanged. Fiber helps us feel more full and more satisfied because it slows digestion and absorption, allowing sugar (glucose) to enter the bloodstream more slowly. There are two main types of fiber: soluble and insoluble. Soluble fiber dissolves in water and has a positive effect on the body, including lowering bad cholesterol and blood sugar levels. Insoluble fiber cannot be dissolved in water and helps with regularity/elimination. Adult men should aim for a minimum of 38 grams of fiber daily and adult women require a minimum of 25 grams daily. These amounts are based on getting 14 grams of fiber per 1000 calories, as recommended by the Institute of Medicine. For men over fifty, the recommendation decreases to 30 grams daily; and for women over fifty, it goes to 21 grams daily, due to decreased calorie consumption.[2]

Free Range is a marketing term used to describe a method of raising livestock where the animals are permitted to roam freely, as opposed to being contained or restricted. It may also imply but does not assure other meanings, including grass fed, humanely raised, or pasture raised. It is assumed that free-range meats and eggs come from animals allowed to graze on grasses, rather than corn or other grains, but the term is not strictly monitered.

Genetically Modified Organisms (GMOs) are "plants or animals that have been genetically engineered with DNA from bacteria, viruses, or other plants and animals."[3]

Gluten is a starchy wheat protein made up of the proteins gliadin and glutenin, which are present in many mature grass grains, including wheat, rye, barley, kamut, and spelt. It is estimated that approximately 1 percent of the US population has an adverse immune (autoimmune) response to gluten, labeled celiac disease. When individuals with celiac disease eat foods that contain gluten, damage can occur in the small intestine. This can then lead to malabsorption of essential vitamins, minerals, and other nutrients, causing additional health risks. The number of individuals with gluten intolerance or sensitivity is on the rise; some scientists and health researchers attribute part of this to genetically modified (GM) crops, especially GM wheat.

Glycemic Index (GI) is a ranking of foods (from 0 to 100) according to their effect on blood glucose levels. High GI foods (ranking of 70 and above) are quickly digested and can result in wacky blood-sugar fluctuations. Low GI foods (55 and under) are digested and absorbed more slowly, and have been shown to be beneficial to people with both type 1 and type 2 diabetes. Low GI foods also help with weight management and appetite control. Examples of low GI foods include dark-green leafy vegetables (broccoli, cabbage, lettuce, kale); onions; peas; cherries; plums; grapefruit; peaches; apples; pears; coconut; grapes; berries; whole milk; yogurt; legumes; brown rice; wheat tortillas; buckwheat; whole-grain pasta; rolled oats; oat bran; nuts; and seeds. High GI foods include honey, sugar, corn syrup, bananas, white bread, white rice, corn, potato chips, popcorn, rice cakes, beer, melons, pineapples, watermelon, raisins, most cereals, parsnips, and beets.

Greek Yogurt is a thicker, creamier, richer style of yogurt that has higher protein content than most regular yogurts. It is made by straining yogurt until it becomes thick.

Greens or Powdered Greens are generally a powdered form of phytonutrients formulated from foods like fruits, vegetables, seaweeds, herbs, and/or grasses. Nutritional information and taste can vary considerably between greens products; so, look for greens that do not contain artificial sweeteners, colors, or flavoring agents. We love Skoop, designed by Dr. James and available at drdeb.healthyskoop.com.

High-Fructose Corn Syrup (HFCS) is a sweetener to avoid. It is a highly refined, almost always genetically modified sugar that the body doesn't metabolize well. HFCS is added to a wide array of foods (from sweets, breads, and cakes to condiments), and has links to increased rates of obesity. HFCS is made by milling corn to produce cornstarch, which is made into corn syrup (almost total glucose), and then changes into fructose through an additional process. It is often added to foods you wouldn't suspect, so please read ingredients labels.

Hormones are chemical messengers secreted from different glands in the body into the bloodstream, influencing many of the body's functions—mood, metabolism, growth, cognitive function, sexual function, reproduction, and body temperature (to name a few).

Neurotransmitters are brain chemicals that communicate information between nerve cells throughout the body and the brain.

Phytonutrients are chemical-like compounds found in plants that have shown promise in disease prevention. They can be further classified into different antioxidant groupings, including flavonoids, carotenoids, isoflavones, lignans, saponins, and indoles.

Pin Bones are thin, long, floating bones that aren't attached to the main skeleton of a fish. They can be difficult to see, but you'll definitely notice them when you get a mouthful. Even though you choose a fish that has been filleted, pin bones will often remain hidden in the flesh. The best way to find them is to carefully fan your (very clean) fingers over the length of the fillet. Sliding a hand under the fillet may help the bones to protrude and make them easier to remove. The bones themselves are slippery, so you need a tool with a good grip to remove them—something like fish tweezers, which you can find online or at specialty gourmet kitchen stores. Small needlenose pliers are another option.

Polyphenols are chemical compounds found in certain foods that may be beneficial to our health. Polyphenols have antioxidant activity that may reduce the risk of heart disease and certain cancers. Food sources include tea, red wine and grapes, berries, cocoa, walnuts, pomegranates, peanuts, prunes, raisins, blueberries, kale, strawberries, spinach, rasp-berries, Brussels sprouts, plums, broccoli, beets, oranges, red grapes, red bell peppers, and cherries.

Protein, Soy is a popular protein choice among vegans. Soy protein iso-late comes from defatted soy flour that has had most of the nonprotein components, fats, and carbohydrates removed. It contains roughly 90 percent protein by weight. Because of this, it has a neutral flavor and will cause less flatulence due to bacterial fermentation. Soy protein concen-trate preserves much of the fiber of the original soybean, and contains about 70 percent protein. We only recommend organic soy if you choose to use soy products. Both whey and soy protein powders are widely available at most grocery stores and natural food stores. Other forms of protein powder that are available but are sometimes more difficult to find include hemp protein, brown rice protein (and sprouted rice pro-tein), pea protein, and egg white protein.

Protein, Whey is typically available in three major types: concentrate, isolate, and hydrolysate. All offer a very well digested and biologically available protein. Whey protein concentrate contains a fairly low level of fat and cholesterol, lactose, and carbohydrate, and can fluctuate consid-erably in protein content. Whey protein isolate has typically had the fat and lactose removed, and has a higher percentage of protein by weight. Whey protein hydrolysates are the most easily absorbed and least aller-genic varieties of whey protein. Both whey protein concentrate and isolate have a milky flavor, while the hydrolysate form has a more bit-ter taste. Whey protein contains branched chain amino acids (BCAAs), which are used to build and fuel muscles. Whey protein also contains amino acids like cysteine and glutamine, which can be used to synthesize glutathione in the body. Glutathione is a powerful antioxidant that may protect against certain types of cancer.

Quinoa is a higher protein, naturally gluten-free "ancient" seed-grain (and it's really not a grain or a seed but a fruit). There is a natural, bitter saponin residue that coats the seeds, so the quinoa needs to be well rinsed prior to cooking. Quinoa (pronounced keen-wah), is a relative of spinach and Swiss chard that is high in complete protein, magnesium, manganese, iron, tryptophan, and fiber. In most of our recipes calling for quinoa, brown rice may be substituted.

Tamari is Japanese soy sauce made by using traditional brewing methods. It tastes basically the same as soy sauce. We always use San-J Organic Wheat-Free Reduced Sodium Tamari that is a certified gluten-free product.

Teff is a tiny little nutty grain that is high in protein, calcium, and iron. It is found in the form of flour or as a whole grain, and is naturally gluten free.

Tempeh is a soy food made from partially cooked and fermented soybeans. It has high protein content and can be marinated, stir-fried, baked, or stewed. Again, choose organic.

Tofu, also known as bean curd, originated in China and is made by coagulating soy milk. Tofu is a decent source of protein, is high in iron, and usually contains magnesium and calcium, depending on how it was processed. Choose organic tofu when possible.

Trans Fats may occur naturally in meat and dairy products, but they are also produced during the hydrogenation process of oils. Partially hydrogenated oils add shelf life to processed foods, but they also increase the risk or coronary heart disease and metabolic syndrome. Avoid trans fats whenever possible.

GLOSSARY

Tryptophan is an amino acid found in poultry, red meat, eggs, chocolate, oats, dates, mangoes, dried dates, milk, yogurt, cottage cheese, red fish, chickpeas, sunflower seeds, pumpkin seeds, sesame seeds, and peanuts. Tryptophan has been used as a sleep aid and as an antidepressant in mild depression and seasonal affective disorder.